DAILY DOSE
OF TOXINS

by

Dr. Marilyn Chernoff, PhD, ND, M.Ed

Compiled and edited by Kyre Adept, PhD

Note for Librarians: A cataloguing record for this book is available from Library and Archives
Canada at www.collectionscanada.ca/amicus/index-e.html
ISBN 1-4120-6422-8

*Printed in Victoria, BC, Canada. Printed on paper with minimum 30% recycled fibre. Trafford's print shop
runs on "green energy" from solar, wind and other environmentally-friendly power sources.*

TRAFFORD
PUBLISHING™

Offices in Canada, USA, Ireland and UK
This book was published *on-demand* in cooperation with Trafford Publishing. On-demand
publishing is a unique process and service of making a book available for retail sale to the
public taking advantage of on-demand manufacturing and Internet marketing. On-demand
publishing includes promotions, retail sales, manufacturing, order fulfilment, accounting and
collecting royalties on behalf of the author.

Book sales for North America and international:
Trafford Publishing, 6E–2333 Government St.,
Victoria, BC V8T 4P4 CANADA
phone 250 383 6864 (toll-free 1 888 232 4444)
fax 250 383 6804; email to orders@trafford.com
Book sales in Europe:
Trafford Publishing (UK) Ltd., Enterprise House, Wistaston Road Business Centre,
Wistaston Road, Crewe, Cheshire CW2 7RP UNITED KINGDOM
phone 01270 251 396 (local rate 0845 230 9601)
facsimile 01270 254 983; orders.uk@trafford.com
Order online at:
trafford.com/05-1333

10 9 8 7 6 5 4 3 2

ACKNOWLEDGMENTS

With appreciation, I gratefully acknowledge the teaching, published books and concepts of:

- Dr. Devi Nambudripad, creator of NAET

- Rev. Hanna Kroeger, master herbalist

- Dr. John Christopher

- Dr. Hulda Clark

- Dr. Ellen Jensen

- Dr. Bernard Jensen

Without these writers and thinkers, this work and my own research would not have been possible. Any errors of omission, quotation or interpretation are, of course, my own.

I also give heartfelt thanks to my wonderful and supportive husband.

DEDICATION

This book is dedicated to all those people who suffer from the plethora of chemicals that exist in our society today. If this book helps you to better understand what causes you harm, then this book is a success.

For children entering our society, some of the effects of the chemicals we digest, breathe, and put on our bodies will not be known for many years. If this book helps them avoid some of the problems with chemicals and their effects on the body, then this book will serve its purpose.

I want to thank all the people who deliberately or inadvertently gave me clues to the problems they were having. They allowed me to treat them for the chemicals that had affected them.

And special thanks to my wonderful husband who supported my long hours writing and completing this book.

Marilyn Chernoff, PhD, ND, M.Ed

REVIEWS OF *DAILY DOSE OF TOXINS*

Dr. Marilyn Chernoff's book *Daily Dose of Toxins* is a much-needed addition to everyone's bookshelf. We are exposed to a multitude of toxins that adversely affect our immune systems. Dr. Chernoff describes the various toxins and how we can avoid them. Chronic illnesses including cancer, heart disease and autoimmune disorders are occurring at epidemic rates. My clinical experience has shown, beyond a doubt, that exposure to toxic items play a large part in etiology of these illnesses. Dr. Chernoff gives a specific treatment plan, NAET, which helps one's body overcome these toxic items. I believe Dr. Chernoff's treatment plan is ahead of its time. This book is a must-read for all interested in improving their health. I highly recommend this book to not only those suffering from chronic illness but also to practitioners treating chronic illness.

David Brownstein, M.D., www.drbrownstein.com, author of *The Miracle of Natural Hormones*, 3rd Edition, *Overcoming Arthritis, Overcoming Thyroid Disorders* and *Iodine: Why You Need It, Why You Can't Live Without It*

"*Daily Dose of Toxins* is an extensive reference on the source of and symptoms caused by a large number of toxins. It will help energy practitioners understand the broad area of environmental toxicology and help them focus their testing therapies so people can more healthfully live in the "chemical soup" of our modern society.

Jacob Teitelbaum, MD, www.endfatigue.com, author of *From Fatigued to Fantastic* and *Pain Free 1-2-3*

"Toxic environmental pollution is rampant in our society today and the most frequent reason for the onset of chronic degenerative diseases. Since it is virtually impossible to avoid exposure, this book will help to educate and alert us to the symptoms and sources. Congratulations to Dr. Chernoff for her dedication to this important subject. She realized that so many so-called diseases can be traced back to toxic pollution and set out to compile this book to help us to maintain or regain our health in a toxic environment".

Arianne Koven, Traditional Naturopath

Daily Dose of Toxins is timely, concise and practical for healers of all types and the public. Everyone has to be concerned about the welfare of their children, as well as for themselves. This succinct common-sense book accurately describes many aspects related to chemical exposures of which most people are not aware. Too many people have no idea what types of symptoms can be caused by chemicals and many health professionals have not been exposed to this type of illness in their continuing medical education programs. This combination is exceedingly bad because the illness is simply not recognized for what it is. Others have heard about chemical sensitivities but continue to keep their heads in the sand because they don't believe or want to think about what is happening. Better to adopt an empowering approach to handle the challenging situation of harmful effects from toxins. We must all begin to learn how, what, when, where and why so many poisons are confronting and hurting us. The Tables in the latter half of Dr. Chernoff's book are essential to help identify specific chemicals and associated symptoms. The therapies suggested in this book reflect beyond the usual approaches, some definitely being "cutting edge". Vibrational energy healing is a reality, which should provide more definitive answers.

Dr. Doris Rapp, MD, www.drrapp.com, author of *Our Toxic World, A Wake Up Call*

Table of Contents

FOREWORD

by

Dr. Devi S. Nambudripad

All good words travel fast and spread the good news. I am glad to see that is what has been happening to NAET in recent years; its beneficiaries, practitioners, proponents, advocates, and the public at large who all want to simply help people and minimize worldwide sufferings. By writing this book, "Daily Dose of Toxins," Dr. Marilyn Chernoff has made a bold attempt to help all of us to live better through chemistry and has also made it possible to avoid all illnesses arising from chemical toxins.

Without question, lately, many undiagnosed, puzzling illnesses are appearing among unsuspecting patients worldwide. The actual fact is that there are hardly any human diseases or conditions in which chemical or environmental sensitivities are not involved either directly or indirectly. Potentially, you can be sensitive to anything you come in contact with. If you begin to check people around you – even so-called healthy people – you will find hidden chemical and environmental sensitivities as a causative factor in almost all health problems.

For those whose lives are merely disrupted by the discomfort of the chemical reaction, traditional treatments with simple antihistamine or topical remedies can bring relief. But for more serious sufferers, long-term complete avoidance is the only way to help them reduce their symptoms. Most people finally resort to a lifetime of depriving themselves of the many things in life that would otherwise bring them joy and fulfillment. Common complaints are, *"My sensitivities have taken control of my life,"* and *"The very things that I want to make me happy are the very things that I react to the most."*

Even with avoidance, there is no guarantee that hypersensitive persons will be able to stay away from every situation and still remain reaction free. With the progress of science and technology, our life-styles have changed dramatically. New chemical products, which are potential allergens for many people, are being developed every day. The quality of life has improved; however, for some sensitive patients the scientific achievements have created more nightmares.

We cannot ignore the fact that we are in the 21st century where technology is ever more predominant than before. There is nothing wrong with the technology. In fact, modern technology has provided a better quality of life. But the allergic patient must find ways to overcome adverse reactions to chemicals and other allergens produced by the technology in order to enjoy this world.

We have chosen to live in this world of chemicals by breathing, touching and consuming. However sensitive you may be, now there is no way out of this chosen path. Our genes that came from our simple, ancestors were not quite ready for this sudden, chemical explosion. If we had time to prepare for this situation, our genes would have handled it differently. Our genes have the capabilities to adapt to any situation happily and comfortably if given enough time.

But unfortunately we didn't get enough time to wake up our adaptation skills. More and more, the whole world has been taken over by chemicals... the competitive scientists didn't waste any time...they became extremely industrious to display their scientific achievements in the world market. They did not have any notion that these very chemicals could lead many to their misery some day. At this very time perhaps, the creators of these chemicals do not suffer from any chemical sensitivities or they do not know the symptoms, if they do suffer now, are related to their own inventions. In any case the short term effects are not crippling them. They do not care about the long term effects as long as their products will be most efficient now and during their competitive race, the small percentage of multiple chemical sensitivity (MCS) victims are ignored.

Many people, including some health professionals, upon hearing the word "chemical sensitivity" think only of a runny nose, itching of the eyes, or throat, skin rashes and, perhaps, some hay-fever like symptoms. Yes, the reactions of some allergy sufferers fall into these categories. But for others, the reactions are not at all what would be expected. Their reactions vary radically and appear unexpectedly, making diagnosis elusive and pretreatments nearly impossible. Curiously, although they previously resisted, increasing numbers of medical doctors and researchers are now considering chemical sensitivities and environmental sensitivities in most illnesses and medical disorders.

Multiple Chemical Sensitivity Syndrome patients often suffer from chronic, recurring physical, physiological and psychological illnesses without identifying any specific cause or event. Their symptoms may be caused by a person's inability to tolerate an environmental chemical or man-made chemicals. For years, mainstream medicine refused to recognize or support persons with Multiple Chemical Sensitivities (MCS), which is gradually gaining the recognition that has been overdue. Until recent times, there was no treatment for MCS. People were afraid to tell others about their symptoms, other more fortunate and healthy ones made fun of these victims or teased them and their physicians referred them to psychiatric care and management. For the fear of facing such traumatic events or being ridiculed by the not-so understanding public, these people suffered silently.

But now thanks for the Internet and many public communication services and MCS support groups, more and more patients are coming forward to share and learn from each other and thus the syndrome is being recognized and actually gaining certain legitimacy. The U.S. Department of Housing and Urban Development now considers it a disability under law and Social Security will consider it, on a case-by-case basis. Nonetheless, MCS remains still a mystery and a nuisance to the sufferers. There is no specific test to detect it. If once detected, the person can receive freedom or reduction from the symptoms through NAET (Nambudripad's Allergy Elimination Techniques). But availability of NAET is limited to a small percentage of people now since it is not yet a widely accepted treatment method for sensitivities. Avoidance is the only accepted solution so far, but there is no way for its sufferers to completely avoid the tens of thousands of chemicals in our daily life, especially those hidden chemicals. In fact, where will you look for them and how will you find them?

Thanks to Marilyn for writing this book and asking me to write this foreword and let me highlight the important points that Marilyn wants all of us to take home from this book. For example, what is a multiple chemical sensitivity? The article by Cullin, M.R. ed. (1987) "Workers with multiple chemical sensitivities" *Occupational Medicine; State of the Art Reviews*, defines multiple chemical sensitivity (MCS) as an acquired disorder characterized by recurrent symptoms referable to multiple organ systems, occurring in response to demonstrable exposure to many chemically unrelated compounds at doses far below those established in the general population to cause harmful effects. No single widely accepted test of physiological function can be shown to correlate with these symptoms. [Cullen, M.R. (1987), The worker with multiple chemical sensitivities: an overview, in Cullen, M.R. (Ed). *Occupational Medicine: State of the Art Reviews*, Hanley and Belfus, Philadelphia. 655-662].

Several years ago a committee of experts in the field decided upon a consensus as to what "qualifies" the patient as truly having chemical or environmental sensitivities and illnesses arising from such sensitivities. [Arch Environ Health 1999; 54: 147]. Six criteria were decided upon:

- Symptoms are reproducible with repeated (chemical) exposures.

- The condition is chronic.

- Low levels of exposure (lower than previously or commonly tolerated) result in manifestations of the syndrome (i.e. increased sensitivity).

- The symptoms improve, or resolve completely, when the triggering chemicals are removed.

- Responses often occur to multiple chemically-unrelated substances.

- Symptoms involve multiple-organ symptoms (runny nose, itchy eyes, headache, scratchy throat, ear ache, scalp pain, mental confusion or sleepiness, palpitations of the heart, upset stomach, nausea and/or diarrhea, abdominal cramping, aching joints).

Several other medical conditions appear to be related to, or overlap with, Multiple Chemical Sensitivity Syndromes – such as food intolerance syndrome, food allergies, attention deficit hyperactive disorders, autistic behaviors, learning disability, chronic fatigue syndrome, fibromyalgia, irritable bowel syndrome, lupus arthritis, other joint disorders, asthma and other respiratory disorders, autoimmune disorders, sick-building syndrome, the Gulf War Syndrome, unexplained or idiopathic pain syndrome, drug-induced disorders, multiple sclerosis, reflex sympathetic dystrophy (RSD), eye disorders, ear disorders, and the list can go on. In each of these, a chemical appears to precipitate the symptoms. The immediate trigger may be chemicals in a new rug, house cleaning chemical, water chemical from the city water, cosmetic chemicals, animal dander, formaldehyde in building materials, fabrics, and other vinyl products, chemicals in foods as food additives, food colorings, processed foods, sugar products, pesticides used in spraying on city trees, grasses and bushes, living near a toxic waste dump site, and heavy metal toxins.

[In this situation, cellular processes regulated by the aryl hydrocarbon receptor (AHR) apparently activate an inflammatory response involving TH2 helper cells, subsequently increasing immunoglobulin E (IgE) production.]

In her latest book *Our Toxic World: A Wake Up Call,* Dr. Doris Rapp has tried to explore almost all hidden chemical sources in the world and has a comprehensive description of environmental chemicals and how to minimize your exposure. Information about every study or investigation or experiment ever conducted anywhere in the world on chemicals and sensitivities can be found in her book.

In this book, Dr. Chernoff has tried to inform you about the possible encounters with hidden chemicals in your daily life. This book is very informative for the chemically sensitive person, especially if you do not know where you are getting your daily dose of toxins from. In fact, through this valuable and informative book, Dr. Chernoff is helping us all to become smarter sleuths so that we can try to live a better life. This book is certainly an eye-opener.

Devi S. Nambudripad, M.D., D.C., L.Ac., Ph.D.
Buena Park, California

"Disease is born of like things, and by the attack of like things people are healed."

Hippocrates

Outstanding Symptoms of Toxins

fever	profuse sweating
hypothermia	jaundice
photosensitization	facial paralysis
asthma	pulmonary irritants
eczema	tachycardia
pigmentation	herpes zoster
loss of hair	arteriosclerosis
lupus	corneal damage
hypertension	constipation
insomnia	cataracts
gastroenteritis	pancreatitis
nasal ulcers	tremors
dementia	kidney and bladder issues
impotence	acidosis
pneumonia	vasoconstriction
dysmenorrhea	dryness of the mouth
anemia	diarrhea
acute arthritis	ventricular fibrillation
leukemia	cancer

TOXICITY TODAY

This book discusses the impact of toxins on the physical body, with a view to assisting practitioners in their work of restoring homeostatic balance through detoxification and vibrational healing. Our intention here is three-fold:

1. Providing a brief overview of how toxicity occurs;

2. Giving new knowledge and insight into the toxic effect of even relatively low levels of exposure to various contaminants;

3. Providing practitioners with information about the symptoms and sources of toxic contamination, so that they can better assist their clients/patients to renewed health.

Although the current levels and effects of toxic contamination create a depressing picture, there is good news as well. After all, we see these effects in the increase of asthma, allergies, and auto-immune disorders, as well as a variety of other, "undiagnosable" conditions. Fortunately, advances in vibrational medicine are often able to address these issues quickly and efficiently, frequently releasing patients/clients from years of unspecified weakness and illness.

Toxic contamination

It has long been known that external contaminations can upset our physical systems and create all manner of problems. It's easy to see the more obvious and extreme forms of toxicity, such as swallowing known poisons. After all, many bottles and jars are explicitly labeled as poisonous, and there is a body of folklore regarding the fatal effects of such naturally occurring poisons as hemlock, yew berries, and various mushrooms.

Less obvious are the subtler effects of many manmade toxins, and the potential impact of various foods and other allergens on the human immune system. We see the evidence of increasing toxicity in the mounting incidence of immune system disorders, allergies, birth defects and genetic mutation.

Why do we see more of these conditions than in the past? There are several interlocking factors: people's immune systems are more fragile due to stress and allergens, the quality of nutrition has declined, and there are many more toxic chemicals in the environment, both in quantity and quality.

In terms of impact on the human body, there is a significant difference between natural contaminants and artificial, manmade contaminants. The challenge of synthetic chemicals is that, unlike foods or other naturally produced substances, the human body doesn't recognize them as legitimate substances. The body simply doesn't know how to deal with certain chemical structures, so it will react to them the way a computer reacts to computer viruses. Once introduced into an electronic system, a computer virus will have three possible effects: the computer will crash, it will run a program it doesn't want to, or it will use up system resources to get around the virus. The only way a viral scan program can work is to either isolate or destroy the virus, and the first step to doing that is to recognize what is part of the legitimate system and what is not.

In the same way, a toxin acts as an irritant, and the immune system can only respond by attempting to isolate and/or destroy the toxin. Once this happens, the immune system has a "file" on that toxin and will automatically attack it once the presence of the particular toxin is detected; this usually results in allergies and/or detectable antibodies. Sometimes the immune system is too weak to prevail against the toxin, and the body succumbs to illness or even death. In other circumstances, a given immune system may be stronger than the contaminant, yet still use up much of the body's vitality in combating or avoiding the effects of a poison. In many cases, the immune system is compromised, even if no overt symptoms are detected. It doesn't take many such contaminations to have a lasting effect on the body's overall health and vitality.

If we define a toxin as any external, chemical substance that distorts the correct internal functioning of the body, there are five basic types of toxins:

1. Natural substances such as elements, foods, herbs, molds, and pathogens

2. Medicinal drugs, chemotherapy and radiation, with iatrogenic effects

3. Pesticides and other agricultural chemicals

4. Petrochemicals, including dyes, plastics, and cleaning products

5. Other "accidental" environmental toxins, such as xeno-estrogens

People can develop allergies and other sensitivities to any or all of these contaminants. Although we will be focusing on synthetic or manmade toxins, a system already weakened by stress, poor nutrition, congenital weakness, or environmental hazards will also be more susceptible to natural contaminations, or may experience otherwise healthy foods, herbs, or elements as allergenic.

At times, the ingestion process becomes a cycle that draws all factors into a deepening spiral. For instance, Elizabeth Weise recently wrote the following in *USA Today*:

> *The chemical compounds that keep our leftovers fresh and make our floors easy to clean may be a factor in the rising levels of asthma and allergies in children around the world over the past 30 years.*
>
> *Five million U.S. children have asthma and 10%-20% of infants have eczema, the Asthma and Allergy Foundation of America reports. The Centers for Disease Control and Prevention estimates the cost of treating asthma in these children at $3.2 billion per year.*
>
> *An extensive study of Swedish children found that house dust containing the softeners in plastic that give flexibility to food containers, vinyl floor tiles and cling wrap is associated with higher rates of asthma, eczema and other allergy symptoms. The compounds, phthalates, are widely used in moisturizers, nail polish, insect repellants, shower curtains, hairsprays and building products such as polyvinyl chloride flooring.*
>
> *Because they leach out of products, they are considered ubiquitous environmental contaminants. Global phthalate production is 3.8 million tons per year. "We've*

measured lots of things and there are no other factors that have shown this kind of raised risk," says Carl-Gustaf Bornehag of the Swedish National Testing and Research Institute, lead study author.

While Bornehag says the research doesn't contain enough evidence "to make us recommend that parents throw out everything that's plastic in their home," he called for serious and rapid research to confirm the findings.

The American Chemistry Council notes that it's hard to tell whether phthalates are the cause of the children's asthma, or an effect. "It is common practice to replace carpeting with smooth, easy-to-clean surfaces, such as vinyl, in the homes of children suffering from asthma, in order to reduce dust," the council's Marian Stanley says. "So the question is, do the children have asthma because of the vinyl on the floor, or is there vinyl on the floor because they have asthma?"

Indeed, in the case of autoimmune conditions, the body interprets some part of its own system as "foreign", and therefore depletes itself in attacking its own native substance. One factor in the vast recent increase in autoimmune diseases lies in the confusion caused as the immune system attempts to classify and deal with synthetic substances that fall outside its natural recognition programs. It's as if these synthetic substances are new computer viruses that the body's viral scanning system doesn't know to recognize and therefore cannot deal with adequately.

The more complex the chemical, the more likely it is to set up negative immune system responses. This is another reason for the rapid proliferation of immune system complaints caused by manmade chemicals. Some of these recently created chemicals have more complex structures than nature could have produced, and again, the immune system doesn't know how to cope with them. It's the same with radioactive substances. In the dilute conditions in which they are found in nature, radioactive elements are relatively harmless; it's only when humans gather together unnatural quantities and purify them into "usable" forms that radioactive materials become poisonous. After 50 years, we are only beginning to understand the long-term impact of radioactive elements on the human immune system. It is becoming increasingly clear that other synthetic toxins may have equally damaging long-term effects.

Finally, we need to keep in mind that toxins can affect us on both physical and nonphysical (i.e., energetic) levels. Physical contaminations and symptoms are, of course, easier to quantify; however, energetic contaminations can be dealt with more easily and quickly than conditions that have already manifested into physical symptoms. The toxin checklists in this book can be used as to clear people in the energy fields as well as on a physical level.

Before we get to those checklists, however, we present an overview of how toxins get into the body, ways their presence can affect the human system, and ways they leave the body. Of course, with such a wide variety of toxic chemicals currently in the world it is impossible to cover each of them in detail. We seek simply to remind readers of the overall mechanisms of toxic contamination, and the general principles of how to avoid and/or release contamination once it is present.

TOXINS IN THE BODY

We talk about being poisoned by this or that, and have the picture of someone swallowing strychnine or prussic acid and collapsing on the spot. In fact, most toxicity is much more subtle – yet more far-reaching – in its effects. We live surrounded by chemicals that we eat and drink, breathe or touch. Toxins make their way into our systems as frequently through our lungs and skins as they do through our stomachs. We need to understand the whole mechanism of how toxins affect us – ingestion, processing and excretion – in order to see how to deal with their effects on physical health.

So how do toxins get into the system? There are four basic ways to pass the boundaries between *in here* and *out there*:

1. Breathed in through the lungs and other mucus membranes via exposure to the nose, eyes, etc.

2. Ingested through the alimentary canal via ingestion by mouth, affecting stomach, intestines

3. Through the skin, via direct exposure to toxic liquids or gases

4. Directly into the bloodstream via injection, as with medication or drugs

It's not always obvious how a particular substance comes into a person's system. For example, a caustic liquid may burn the skin, yet the real damage can be done to the lungs as the person inhales the vapors, damaging the lung surfaces and releasing toxins into the bloodstream. However, one way or another, these contaminations always end up in the bloodstream.

Once in the bloodstream, a toxin can go anywhere in the body. However, a given chemical normally has an affinity to a certain organ, system or meridian. Conversely, each organ is vulnerable to certain types of chemicals. These "target organs" are not necessarily the location of the highest concentrations of a given toxin; however, it will be where that toxin can do the most damage. The concentration of a given contaminant in the target organ depends primarily on whether it is introduced by breathing, swallowing or skin contact. Some toxins have more impact when inhaled than when taken in by mouth; others cannot be absorbed from the GI tract, but may lodge in the lungs. Some toxins have less effect on the liver if already diluted by coming through the skin into the bloodstream.

Upper respiratory system

It is vital to understand the effects of toxins coming into the upper respiratory system (URS). We often notice the beginning stages of chemical contamination or sensitivity when the client or patient presents with symptoms to the ear, nose or throat. If the toxic effect is detected and released at an early stage, later and more serious ailments may be prevented altogether.

When a person has symptoms that resemble colds or flu, there is always a temptation to use remedies that suppress the symptoms, as this can be easier than addressing the causes. However, such an approach leaves the patient or client to clog up their immune system with accumulated toxins, leading to more problems on a deeper level later in life. Given that medical treatments often leave the core challenge in place where it can make mischief later, it is better to use such remedies only as a last resort. Further, covering up such ailments may mean that the true significance of the dysfunction is not spotted until further, more chronic, symptoms emerge.

In fact, many ear, nose and throat symptoms can be addressed with relatively simple remedies, such as allergy elimination techniques, nutrition that focuses on organic foods and eliminates food additives, rotation diets, environmental controls, herbal formulations and nutritional supplements. Given that so many effective modalities are easier on the physical system, pharmaceutical suppression of symptoms should only be used as a last resort, especially as covering up symptoms with medication can allow relatively minor ailments to result in the spread of immune system sensitivity and other possible damage to target organs. This is a particular concern for inflammatory diseases, many of which are either triggered or exacerbated by increasing sensitivity to allergens or chemical toxins.

Because this is a frequent entry point for more serious conditions, any symptoms to the ear, nose or throat should be screened for environmental, nutritional and allergic factors and triggers. This section described the effects of toxins that come in through the ear, nose or throat to affect the upper respiratory tract. The checklists that make up the second part of the book can be used to ascertain which toxins are involved in a particular contamination; in this section we will also make some suggestions as to how to contain such contaminations once the patient/client has been exposed to them.

The Nose

If a person is sensitive to chemicals or allergies, the nose is often the first place the contamination is experienced. As well as affecting the nose itself, pollutants can use the nose as the entry point for the nervous system, blood system, sinuses and sense of smell.

The **lymph system** has connections to the nose in both anterior and posterior networks. The anterior network of lymph nodes and vessels drain along the facial muscles to empty in the neck. Because this anterior network is connected to the front part of the nose, it is where a person can show the first signs of allergic or chemical sensitivity.

The posterior network is larger, and connects the three main channels in the middle and back part of the nose to the retrolaryngeal nodes, the jugular nodes, and other lymph nodes in the neck. Toxins and/or allergens can enter through any of these channels and cause local symptoms like crying, regional conditions such as inflammation, and/or systemic conditions throughout the body. The first sign of environmental toxicity is often observable and chronic swelling in the lymph nodes along in the neck. If this is a frequently observed phenomenon, there may well be triggering agents that should be identified and neutralized.

The lymph nodes are the part of the neck most frequently affected by pain and swelling. This can be triggered by foods, food additives, or environmental toxins. Symptoms can include sore throats, tonsillitis, and difficulty in swallowing, sometimes immediately after exposure. The nodes may swell and remain swollen for weeks, knocking out the immune system, thus increasing the person's vulnerability to pathogens like viruses and bacteria.

Other environmental toxins can affect the posterior nodes, causing swelling to the posterior lymph nodes, stiff necks, muscle spasms and/or headaches. At times, these headaches can be misdiagnosed as tension headaches. Again, this type of swelling can last for weeks after the initial contamination or exposure. Detective work and muscle testing may be needed to determine the original source. On the plus side, avoiding or neutralizing the allergen or toxin may lead to rapid relief of immediate symptom and the avoidance of eventual systemic toxicity.

If the **nerve supply** to the nose is damaged by environmental exposure, it can lead to either greater or lesser sensitivity to smells. In turn, this can affect the sense of taste. Because autonomic control of the sense of smell is regulated by the sympathetic and parasympathetic fibers in the nose, damage to these nerves can lead to immediate or later distortion of the olfactory functions. Chemical and other environmental toxicity can frequently be detected first in this type of symptom.

Because the olfactory neurons are the only part of the central nervous system to reach the actual surface of the body, these neurons are especially vulnerable to environmental contamination; this may be one reason why we frequently see a connection between damage to both the autonomic and nonautonomic nervous system dysfunctions caused by exposure to environmental toxins.

The olfactory nerves are also connected to the limbic system and the central axis that includes the pituitary, pineal, hypothalamus, thyroid, pancreas and adrenal glands. It is quite common for a chemically sensitive individual to complain of pain in the sinuses, limbic system, and portions of the brain associated with the hypothalamus. As well as acute or chronic pain, a person with chemical sensitivities may have a hyper-acute or distorted sense of smell. This is because the normal range of ability to register smells – that is, how much it takes for a given scent to be detected – can be affected adversely by an already overloaded nervous system.

This type of over sensitivity with respect to chemicals, fabrics, petroleum products, engine emissions and perfumes is one of the first and clearest signs of overall chemical sensitivity. A frequent pattern is that immediately after the exposure, the person's olfactory system shuts down (de-adaptation) for 3–9 days, followed by hyper-acuity as the cilia regenerate after exposure. Depending on the particular toxin involved, the effects can travel up the olfactory nerve to the hypothalamus, causing repercussions throughout the brain and the nervous system. This can happen quite rapidly, within minutes after exposure; alternatively, it can take quite a long time to see or measure the effects on the brain or nervous system.

We see this most often when a person starts sneezing after exposure to food, chemicals, or other environmental toxins. Sometimes such reactions last for 10 seconds, sometimes for nine or ten hours. Reaction times depend on how the strength and duration of the exposure and how sensitive and/or overloaded the person's system may already be. Cumulative toxicity leads to increased sensitivity in the nose and is a further indicator of the possibility of organ damage. We see this repeated pattern when looking at prolonged exposure to specific occupational industrial toxins, such as petroleum, phosphorus, or nickel.

Toxic exposure has been shown to lead to degeneration of the mucus membranes as well as inflammation and hyper-acuity. Presenting symptoms can include in sneezing, coughing, polyps, and/or sinusitis. Eventual immune system involvement can be seen in fever, myalgia, and general malaise.

Throat and larynx

Sore throats are very common in chemically sensitive persons, especially during seasons of high dust, pollen or mold counts. Chronic sore throats often indicate food or environmental allergies and toxins, especially from tobacco in any form, carbolic acid, formaldehyde (from furniture), pesticides (from food or air), or chlorine (from town water supplies).

Another way in which the neck can be affected by exposure to toxins is carotodynia, which means pain, spasm, and/or inflammation of the carotid artery. This is frequently a result of an immune system response to being exposed to food or chemical toxins. Fortunately, in most cases, the toxic response will normally disappear when exposure is eliminated.

With respect to the larynx, toxic contamination can result in temporary or permanent hoarseness, spasm, croup (in children), leukoplakia, edema, aphonia, and new tissue growth. As with other types of toxic contamination, the presenting symptoms can be cleared up relatively quickly; however, if ignored or overlooked, such initial exposures can lead to serious long-term consequences in terms of end-organ disorders.

Ingestion through breathing

If a chemical enters through breathing, the rate of absorption depends on factors like the size of the molecule, whether it is water or fat soluble, and the breathing pattern at the time. Some water-soluble contaminants are dissolved quickly enough by the mucus membranes that they never make it to the deep recesses of the lungs. However, fat-soluble chemicals usually do reach the alveoli, where they rapidly get absorbed into the bloodstream. This is particularly true of the smaller-sized particles, although these sometimes get trapped in the alveoli, leading to conditions like silicosis and asbestosis.

Large particles tend to get trapped in the nasal hairs and are later expelled by coughing, sneezing, or swallowing. If swallowed, they act like other swallowed particles, with the same track as food or other ingested contaminants.

Clearly, the level of breathing is a major factor in how much of a given air-borne chemical will be brought into the body. Deep breathing after exercise is bound to result in more contamination than shallow breathing by a person who is sitting or relaxing. Children breathe more frequently and deeply than adults, and therefore will receive more exposure per pound of body weight.

The fact that ingestion is through the lungs does not, in itself, mean that the lungs are the target organ. In fact, many industrial contaminants create more damage in the liver or kidneys than in the lungs. The greatest impact to the lungs is created by caustic fumes that burn the lung surfaces, or particulates such as asbestos or silicon that lodge in the inner recesses of the lungs and cannot be expelled.

Ingestion by mouth

Once swallowed, poisonous chemicals are absorbed slowly or quickly depending upon the state of the gastrointestinal tract. This in turn reflects overall GI health, the time elapsed since the last meal, and the overall speed of an individual's metabolism. Some substances are absorbed quickly from the GI tract, such as alcohol; others cannot be absorbed at all, and thus pass out of the body through urine or feces. Anything absorbed by the digestive system passes through the liver on its way to the bloodstream, and therefore chemicals that target the liver are particularly dangerous when ingested by mouth.

Large quantities of toxic chemicals tend to overload the system in a different way than smaller quantities. Although smaller quantities can be transformed by the liver on their way to the blood stream, larger quantities may go directly to the blood stream without passing through the liver. Thus ingestion by mouth may lead to less toxic effects than absorption through the skin or lungs, as the latter absorption must always be filtered through the kidneys or liver on its way to the blood stream.

Because ingestion by mouth and consequent absorption by the GI tract is a relatively slow process, some *acute* toxins can be removed by stomach pump, enema, or induced vomiting. Smaller doses given long term cannot be removed by these methods; such toxins must pass out of the body naturally. The faster the metabolism, helped by a diet full of fiber and water, the more quickly toxic chemicals will pass through and out of the system.

Ingestion through the skin

Although intact skin is an excellent barrier against most types of contamination, certain caustic and toxic substances are able to penetrate the epidermal layers directly (as well as the toxins that can enter easily through skin cuts, nicks or burns). As the skin has an ample blood supply close to the surface, toxins that do get through the skin go quickly into the blood and are rapidly carried throughout the body. Again, the fact that a toxin is readily absorbed does not mean that the skin or even the blood is the target organ for that substance.

Chemicals that affect the skin come in two basic types: those that burn or dissolve the skin itself, and those that affect the entire system through contaminating the blood. Surface contamination can be seen in burns, rashes, and allergic reactions. Irritant chemicals can also cause itching or burning, and can sometimes thicken the skin, as well leading to scaly or cracked skin, thickened finger and toenails, and dull or brittle hair. Other possible symptoms include pigmentation changes, hair loss, lesions, and local rashes and/or inflammation.

Systemic contamination shows itself in inflammation of entire limbs (rather than local patches), general weakening of the immune system and damage to other organs (depending on the target organ(s) involved). One way of detecting chemicals that have got to the bloodstream and other parts is when that toxin is excreted rapidly through the lungs or urine shortly after exposure.

As with other types of ingestion, the rate of absorption depends on factors such as whether the toxic substance is dry or liquid, and water or fat soluble. Liquid, fat soluble chemicals tend to be absorbed more quickly, especially when the skin itself is wet or injured. Certain chemicals make the skin itself more open to contamination. Water-soluble chemicals are easier to wash off the skin or flush from the blood stream, while dry toxins can often be brushed off, and, at minimum, usually need to be dissolved by liquids before entry through the skin.

Processing toxins in the body

Whether they enter by mouth, skin or lungs, virtually all toxins end up in the bloodstream. From there they are distributed throughout the body and especially to the organ that has a particular affinity for that chemical. There are three ways that the body can attenuate the effect of a given toxin: metabolism, binding the toxin to proteins in the blood, and removing it from active circulation by storing it in the body's tissues.

Metabolism refers to the chemical processes that break down food into nutrients and energy, leading to waste products that are then excreted. This complex process starts as soon as the toxin is ingested. Metabolism can often detoxify a chemical by reducing it to its constituent metabolites. However, metabolism can also intensify the impact of certain chemicals through bioactivation. It can be very difficult to discern whether a particular toxic reaction arises directly from the chemical itself or from the metabolized version (i.e., the metabolite). The rate and extent of metabolism is determined by genetic sensitivity, exposure to other chemicals, and any repeated, gradual ingestion leading to increased tolerance of a particular toxin (such as alcohol or arsenic). There is also a relationship between some chemicals and the enzymes required to metabolize that chemical; when the toxin itself knocks out its corresponding enzyme (or if anything else blocks this enzyme, such as genetic mutation), then this can eliminate the body's ability to deal with a particular toxin.

Binding to proteins is a process of chemical connection between specified chemicals (or their metabolites) and proteins in the blood or organs. The blood itself consists of various blood cells supported by watery plasma that contains salts, trace elements, and protein. Some toxins are chemically attracted to the blood proteins, and these toxic molecules remain in the blood, their larger aggregate size preventing the normal absorption into the organs through the membranes of the blood vessels. Although such toxins have a smaller effect on their target organs, eventually they may detach from their proteins, leading to chronic rather than acute toxic conditions. Also, bioactivation can lead to a stronger level of damage over time than acute poisoning by the unmetabolized toxin. This is frequently the case with carcinogenic chemicals.

Storage occurs when certain chemicals link up with fat particles and are then carried into storage with the fats in relatively safe parts of the body tissues, such as in fat or the bones. On the other hand, if the storage place should be disturbed, such accumulations can leach back into the system. The effects can be quite dangerous, as when (for example) lead is attached to calcium in the bones. As the calcium is used (as in pregnancy or osteoporosis), the lead can be released into the blood, creating delayed lead poisoning. Similarly, weight loss can lead to the release of toxins stored in the body fat. These released toxins will then be attracted to their target organs in the usual way.

Reaching the target organ

The majority of toxins do relatively little damage while in the bloodstream itself; the toxic effect comes when the chemical reaches its target organ after passing through various membranes, such as cell walls, capillary walls, or intestinal walls. The speed and intensity of the toxic effect depends on the characteristics of the chemical and the membrane involved, and on whether the process is passive (i.e., passing through osmotic diffusion) or active (through transmission by "carrier" chemicals).

Certain membranes are intentionally permeable, such as the capillaries in the liver (so that the blood can be cleansed) or in the kidneys (so that water can be reabsorbed). On the other hand, the blood capillaries are tightly sealed so that the brain can be protected from toxic contamination. This constitutes the "blood-brain barrier". The placenta was formerly thought to be "tight" in this sense, but recent research indicates that more toxins may be getting through this membrane than was thought at first. In the same way that we can assume energetic contamination affects the fetus in utero, we must also assume that chemical toxins affect both mother and baby alike. This applies both to the food or environmental toxins to which a pregnant woman is exposed, and also to the toxins released by the changing biological processes that occur during pregnancy.

In general, small water-soluble molecules filter through the membranes by diffusion, which is relatively random in nature. Large water-soluble molecules are too big for diffusion and not amenable to dissolving in fat-based membranes, and therefore a more active chemical process is involved. Because many toxins bear some resemblance to nutrients, the same carriers are involved in their active transport across cell membranes. Thus, the toxins not only have a poisonous effect in their own right, they also "take the seats" of nutrients that would otherwise be nourishing the cells and organs.

Fat-soluble membranes tend to dissolve into the fat-rich membranes and reform on the other side. Many of these membranes are designed to protect organs from water-soluble toxins; however, a fat-based membrane cannot block any fat-soluble toxin from entering. This process works in both directions; even when a fat-soluble toxin reaches a storage location on its way towards excretion, it will frequently be reabsorbed into the bloodstream through the membrane and recycled through the system to do more damage.

Once in the target organ, toxins have a wide variety of effects that come in three basic types: overstimulation, suppression, or distortion of normal function. Again, the type of activity depends on the chemical itself, the nature of the organ affected, and the whether the toxin acts as a catalyst or not. In overstimulation, the toxin generally blocks a governing function that would otherwise be taking place; without natural limiting messages, organs or cells don't know when to stop chemical or growth processes. This is the chief mechanism of toxins that cause cancers. In suppression, the toxic chemical is normally taking the place of a natural part of that organ's processing cycle. Catalytic toxins have the most impact, because they are relatively uninvolved with the chain reaction they cause; at the end of the chemical interaction it causes, such a toxin is able to repeat the process with the next set of matching molecules, and the next, and the next.

Leaving the body

Quite frequently, toxins leave the body the way they came in. An inhaled chemical may be exhaled before reaching the alveoli that would transfer it into the bloodstream. A toxin ingested by mouth might well remain unabsorbed and be excreted after traveling the length of the GI tract. A toxin affecting the skin might be dissolved or washed off before too much damage is done.

However, once a given chemical has made it into the bloodstream, the picture gets more complex. There are three main ways of excreting toxins: through exhalation, urine, and feces. Fat-soluble vapor-based chemicals such as acetone may be exhaled; however, most chemicals are excreted through the urine and feces, which basically means that they pass first through the kidneys or liver, respectively.

The kidneys are vital to removing toxins from the body, as they filter waste products from the blood. During this filtration process, fat-soluble chemicals can easily be reabsorbed into the blood through the membranes, but water-soluble toxins remain in the urine until the latter is released from the body. Therefore, fat-soluble chemicals must be metabolized into water-soluble substances before they can be flushed out with the urine. This is another point in favor of drinking lots of water: as well as assisting kidney function, a properly hydrated system reabsorbs less contaminated water from the kidneys.

Toxins that are primarily processed by the liver exit the body with the feces. Chemicals or their metabolites are transferred by the liver's bile to the gallbladder, and from there to the small intestine. Once within the GI tract, toxins pass to the large intestine, where they are eliminated with the feces. During this trek, there is ample opportunity for fat-soluble toxins to be reabsorbed into the bloodstream, particularly if the person has "leaky gut syndrome". So even if the liver has taken chemicals out of the bloodstream, they may recirculate and pass several times through the liver until they are finally metabolized into water-soluble compounds and finally leave the body. For many people, regular liver cleanses assist the general elimination of toxins from the body.

Although these are the main three ways of ridding the body of toxins, small quantities may also be excreted through sweat or in mother's milk. Sweated toxins may cause skin rashes or other skin sensitivities; we notice this process when large quantities of alcohol, garlic, or fenugreek exude from the skin relatively rapidly after ingestion.

Mother's milk is about 4% fat, so fat-soluble chemicals can easily diffuse into the milk and accumulate there. This can include compounds such as nitrates, DDT and PCBs, as well as toxins that are chemically similar to calcium, such as lead. Since babies are so small and vulnerable as they develop their internal organs and systems, the quantities of such toxins will have a disproportionately large effect on a growing infant. The effects of toxins absorbed in infancy may not show up until middle age, particularly with carcinogens.

Having said this, the benefits of breast-feeding are much greater than the risks. However, for both mother and child, attention to toxic contamination of the mother can make a major difference to the overall health and vitality of the child.

TOXIC SENSITIVITY

There are known acute and chronic effects associated with various toxic chemicals, and these are described by many excellent books, some of which can be found in the attached bibliography (such as John Harte's *Toxics A to Z: A Guide to Everyday Pollution Hazards*). Rather than giving exhaustive descriptions of specific individual toxins and their metabolism, we will focus on what creates hypersensitivity in both sensitive groups and individuals.

Anecdotally and statistically, it is clear to those working in the fields of medicine and allergy prevention that many more people are becoming prone to increased sensitivity to "manmade" chemicals. We see this in vastly increased incidence of autoimmune disease(s), anaphylactic shock, and toxic shock syndrome. Why is it that some people react intensively to allergens and toxins whilst others do not? Why do there seem to be so many more allergies now than previously? And why are so many more people succumbing to systemic immune system ailments, compared to only 50 years ago?

Here we must draw a distinction between sensitivities and allergies. Sensitivity normally affects only the part of the body in contact with the toxin; also, many more people are sensitive to some chemicals than those experiencing true allergies to the same toxin. Allergies will usually affect the entire body. For example, almost every human is sensitive to poison oak, and will normally develop a rash where s/he has come into contact with the plant. A person who is truly allergic may also develop itching eyes, labored breathing and swelling in other parts of the body apart from the actual contact.

An allergy (or, rather, an allergic response) arises from activated antibodies that have previously been sensitized within the bloodstream. Allergy-prone people often seem to inherit more antibodies than others; these antibodies may then get triggered by exposure to specific allergens such as dust, chemicals, foods, etc. (In energy healing work, we also notice that people can develop allergic reactions to other individuals, thoughts, feelings, beliefs, places, and so on.)

Factors in allergy-prone people include genetic predisposition and/or abnormalities, alcohol or drug consumption, the interactions of prescribed drugs, age, pregnancy, and/or the speed and efficiency of metabolism. Some people metabolize more efficiently, while others lack the ability to metabolize certain toxins at all. In general, an inability to metabolize specific chemicals indicates that the person lacks the genetic information to create the necessary enzymes required to deal with that toxin. For example, most adults are unable to create lactase, which breaks down milk sugar (lactose); as a result, the lactose passes undigested into the colon, where it lingers, causing gas, bloating and diarrhea.

There are about 100 similar syndromes that lead to lack of enzymatic metabolism of various proteins, fats, vitamins, or other substances. In some case, this can lead to severe poisoning as there is no way for the body to rid itself even of small doses; in a sensitive individual, these can have as great an impact as much larger amounts might have in a "normal" person. As well as the impact these metabolic conditions have on the body's ability to clear toxins, certain drugs that rely on bioactivation will not work if the enzymes necessary for metabolism are not present.

Another major factor in a person's sensitivity to toxicity is age. Because the physical systems are still developing, a child's enzyme system tends to be more sensitive than an adult's, and a child exposed to carcinogenic materials has longer in which to develop cancer. As most chemically induced cancers take 20-30 years to manifest, such exposure can be a significant additional burden on the immune system. Also, as a person ages, the accumulation of toxins combined with long-term disease or drug use, physical decline, increased or accumulated stress levels and fatigue can make a person react more strongly to specific chemical toxins.

There are lifestyle choices that also affect a person's sensitivity to toxic chemicals, such as lack of exercise, lack of sufficient water, unhealthy diet, smoking or excessive alcohol, the use of medical and recreational drugs, and/or certain diseases such as hepatitis or chronic fatigue syndrome. Certain combinations of lifestyle and contamination are especially lethal; for instance, smoking destroys the cilia in the lungs that are required to move asbestos fibers. Thus, smokers are five times more likely than nonsmokers to develop lung cancer triggered by asbestos. Likewise, alcohol consumption can create faster metabolism with certain chemicals, leading to more toxic impact than if alcohol were not present.

The most central lifestyle choice is probably nutrition. As the quality of the soil declines, the nutritional values of widely available, commercially grown foodstuffs have also taken a nosedive. Thus we absorb fewer nutrients per ounce of a given food than we would have 50 or even 20 years ago. Meanwhile, chemical fertilizers and growth hormones (before processing) and additives (during processing) add considerably to the load of artificial chemicals we ingest and accumulate.

The quality of the food we eat is only one factor in nourishing the body. Leaving aside the toxic contamination of modern foods, the sheer quantity of refined sugars, fats, and carbohydrates consumed by the average American is enough to overwhelm all but the most robust of immune systems. Four ounces of sugar will diminish immune system response by 50%, and the average American consumes 62 *pounds* of sugar per year. Similarly, refined carbohydrates wreak havoc on the digestive tract, encouraging obesity and inhibiting proper digestion and detoxification. For many, saturated fats take the place of essential fatty acids in the cell walls and in the brain, leading to disorders of the circulatory system, skin, nervous system, memory, and attention. Some nutritionists would also argue that meat is toxic to the human system, and certainly the excessive amount of meat consumed by Americans (and the increasing amount of hormones and other chemicals used in its production) adds to the national tendency to obesity, colon cancer, and other digestive ills.

Although simply switching to a diet of organically grown foods with a stronger emphasis on fruits and vegetables will relieve much of the strain on the physical systems, diet alone does not deal with the vast array of chemicals that still surround us. In recent years, some individuals have developed allergies to virtually every manmade substance; such people have to live in "clean rooms" or in the desert, wearing 100% natural fibers without bleaches or dyes, and so on, simply to relieve overtaxed immune systems. Some people even test as allergic to water! What is producing this hypersensitivity now, when it was completely unknown 100 years ago?

One reason is the vast increase in artificial toxins that can be found in the air, soil, water and virtually all the foods we eat. Since the industrial revolution, there has been a tremendous development of new chemical compounds, and only recently have we seen any attempt to curtail their free flow into the environment. Unfortunately, as legal emissions controls have been created, so have even more complex compounds; our awareness of toxicity barely keeps up with the new toxins being created every day. The body's systems are not able to identify or metabolize many of these new toxins, and therefore have no way to deal with them.

In the attempt to fight off these manmade contaminants, the immune system will often create antibodies. These in turn are activated when their specific chemical is ingested again. Especially for sensitive people, this means a constant bombardment of toxins and a consequent up-surge in antibodies. Already weakened by stress, poor food, and/or adverse environmental conditions, the overloaded immune system starts to collapse under the additional weight of constant overstimulation. This is one of the reasons people end up with autoimmune disorders – because the body has become so confused about what is foreign and what is not that it starts creating antibodies for biochemicals that are actually produced by the body.

The most conspicuous autoimmune disease right now is, of course, HIV/AIDS. There is good reason to think that AIDS is an artificially created disease (which argues that there must be a vaccine or antidote in existence as well). Whether "natural" or manmade, AIDS is an excellent example of the fatal results of the immune system that is unable to discern correctly what is "foreign" and what is not. It is now believed that the AIDS virus multiples by persuading the immune system that it is part of the body's natural biochemistry; thus, the virus is able to spread without hindrance, destroying the cells that should be fighting the virus itself.

Another type of immune system damage results from vaccinations. In the worthy attempt to eliminate debilitating diseases such as measles, chicken pox, diphtheria and tuberculosis, many people have allowed doctors to introduce 'dead' or altered pathogens to their systems. On the plus side, vaccination programs appear to have been effective in controlling various diseases that were often fatal in the past. For example, the 1919 flu epidemic killed more people in the U.S. and Europe than died in World War I, so a flu vaccine certainly seemed like a good idea at the time.

On the down side, vaccines leave allergic markers that weaken the immune system; furthermore, vaccine damage is transmitted genetically, and is therefore found in children whose parents were vaccinated, even if the kids were not. Once in the immune system, vaccines combine with viruses, pliomorphs, and other physical or energetic entities to create new pathogens. These morphic constructs are often at the root of ailments that are difficult to diagnose and therefore almost impossible to treat.

Any of these conditions can strip the immune system of its ability to deal with external toxins and internal imbalance. Combine natural resistance with stress, poor diet, and allergic reactions, and the person will sometimes develop hypersensitive reactions to a variety of substances.

CHEMICAL SENSITIVITY SYNDROME

What does it mean to be chemically sensitive? As well as the toxic effects experienced by all humans following exposure to certain chemicals or poisons, certain people have a greatly enhanced level of sensitivity to chemicals in general or specific toxins. Such people can react to a toxic or lethal dose far lower than is considered normal for human exposure. No one really knows why a certain person is sensitive in this way, although it may tie in with a general susceptibility to allergies, which in turn may be genetically linked; on the other hand, we are seeing more cases resulting from toxic contamination itself.

As well as being sensitive in general, the person may also be unable to detoxify a particular chemical because s/he lacks the genetic ability to create the enzyme required to break down or metabolize that particular chemical. Being unable to rid itself of the toxin through metabolism, the body is forced to either store or excrete it. Obviously excretion is more beneficial, and this is why detox techniques are a good choice, where available. With storage, typically in bones or fat, the toxin may emerge years later to spark or add to physical ailments.

With chemical sensitivities, the brain is the primary target. Toxic chemicals tend to be deposited in fat cells, and the brain has a very high fat content (which is one of the reasons that we require essential fatty acids to maintain memory and learning abilities). Smooth muscles are also greatly affected by food and chemical sensitivities. However, chronic symptoms and illness combined with various environmental elements can affect any system or organ of the body, depending on the specific toxin and the weak points of a person's constitution.

Presenting symptoms to the brain can include the following:

- Depression
- Anger
- "Brain fog"
- Emotional instability
- Lightheadedness
- Premature dementia

- Confusion
- Inability to remember or concentrate
- Apathy
- Mental fatigue
- Lethargy
- Loss of cognitive ability

Whether chronic or acute, extreme cerebral reactions can result in psychosis, regression, delusions, disorientation, hallucinations, and/or amnesia. The link between physical toxic contamination and mental/emotional condition is not always obvious or clear-cut.

Neurological response(s) to chemical contamination can include

- Headaches and neck aches
- Nerve pain
- Fainting
- Numbness

- Muscle pain, especially in the chest
- Arthritis
- Restlessness in legs
- Loss or lack of balance

Chemically sensitive people often have an extremely acute sense of smell and are more aware of odors and chemicals than those unaffected. However, individuals may not detect the very chemical or odor that is triggering a reaction. When exposed to chemicals, sensitive people should always breathe through their mouths since chemical fumes entering the nose can directly affect the brain through the bloodstream and pass through the blood-brain barrier before affecting the brain. Ear, nose and throat reactions may involve

- Ringing in the ears
- Cough
- Hypersensitivity to noise
- Nasal obstruction

- Dizziness
- Itching, especially inside the ears
- Rhinitis
- Runny or stuffy nose

After inhalation, the respiratory tract may exhibit symptoms of chemical contamination, including:

- Coughing
- Asthma
- Pulmonary edema

- Bronchitis
- "Air hunger"
- Various sorts of fibrosis

As the most exposed of the mucus membranes, the eyes seem particularly sensitive to chemical contaminations. Symptoms can include:

- Vision disturbances
- Light sensitivity
- Swelling around eyes

- Watery eyes
- Eye pain
- Drooping/swollen/red eyelids

As well as producing the direct symptoms listed below, skin contact can also lead to ingestion, passage into the blood stream, and subsequent organ contamination. Depending on the toxin, any target can be affected, with a variety of symptoms. Unless the skin exposure is very obvious, it may not be possible to trace the path of toxicity from skin to target organ. Meanwhile, direct contamination may be seen in the following:

- Hives
- Blisters
- Itching
- Rashes

- Acne
- Eczema
- Burning
- Caustic burns

Chemical reactions can also have cardiovascular effects, including those from iatrogenic medical drugs. Dr. William Rea has shown in studies on non-atherosclerotic patients that angina symptoms can be triggered by exposure to various chemicals. Other cardiovascular symptoms include the following:

- Heart pounding or racing
- Edema
- Flushing or pallor
- Purpura (hemorrhaging under the skin)

- Palpitations and/or arrhythmia
- Fainting
- Phlebitis (vein inflammation)
- Cardiac arrest

Chemical sensitivity in the gastro-intestinal tract can be seen in the following symptoms:

- Excessive thirst, eating or drinking
- Constipation
- Urgent or frequent urination
- Dry mouth
- Abdominal pain
- Heartburn

- Binges
- Diarrhea
- Nausea/vomiting
- Bad or metallic taste in mouth
- Difficulty in swallowing
- Gallbladder symptoms

Finally, chemically sensitive people can experience musculoskeletal symptoms, such as fatigue, muscle or joint pain, cramps, muscular weakness, stiffness, or lack of coordination.

Chemically susceptible people can be masked to chemicals, just as others can be masked to food allergies. That is, such individuals may not notice what is setting off their symptoms because the exposure may be too familiar. For example, sensitive persons can always identify a fresh paint smell as a problem, because it is not often encountered, but they may not recognize that the odor from a gas range is problematic because they are exposed to it daily and have become masked. If they avoid all natural gas exposures for four to seven days, symptoms will appear upon their return to the natural gas sources because the acquired "normality" has been restored to a contrast condition. This condition is one of the reasons that people are often surprised when their food allergies are diagnosed, while nutritionists know from experience that there is a frequent overlap between allergies and cravings. Often a food craving indicates that the body requires a nutrient that the person is unable to metabolize, whether through transposition (i.e., some other similar chemical taking the nutrient's place on the receptors), through allergic reaction, or through innate inability to create the enzymes required.

Chemically sensitive people can suffer a lifetime of impaired health unless they find proper diagnosis and treatment. They often become unable to work and normal levels of day-to-day comfort can become difficult or even impossible. Fortunately, there are ways of alleviating sensitivities. The main ones are:

- Decreasing exposure to food, chemical, and/or environmental toxins;
- Flushing out existing toxins;
- Increasing immune system response through nutrition and supplements;
- Releasing patterns of toxic sensitivity

We can decrease exposure to contaminants by eating organic foods, drinking pure water, and using air filters or negative ion treatments. Also, chemically sensitive people need to be very careful about the objects they have in their homes and workplaces, as many modern construction materials, paints, cleaners, and furnishings exude toxic fumes. Some carpets and resinous finishes can off-gas for up to three years after manufacture, while many wood preservatives include formaldehyde and other highly toxic chemicals such as pesticides and petrochemicals.

Detoxification is relatively easy with a good diet, plentiful water, and sufficient exercise, especially as there are herbal products and procedures that will target toxins from the colon, liver, kidneys, and so on. Unfortunately, many Americans have chronically blocked colons (and a rising incidence of colon cancer), and this means that toxins are frequently reabsorbed rather than being excreted. Therefore, colonic therapy or cleansing is often recommended before any further detoxification is carried out. Depending on the specific toxic exposure and individual sensitivity, a person will often require detoxification of the liver, kidneys, gall bladder, and/or pancreas. Even the few people who have clear and healthy colons, kidneys, and livers feel the benefit of twice-yearly cleanses. This is one reason that (for example) Gerson Clinics focus on rapid and profound detoxification in order to clear cancers and other serious ailments.

Sluggish immune system response and low-level chronic toxicity often go hand-in-hand. Fortunately, the immune system can be reinforced with proper diet, exercise, lymphatic drainage, herbs, acupuncture and drinking lots of clean water to dilute the lymph fluid. (Water is also essential for flushing toxins, and to allow the cells to process properly on both physical and energetic levels.)

Releasing patterns of allergic/toxic response is possibly the key element to restoring the immune system to its proper level and type of operation. Allergies function like automatic or default computer programs; allergens force a negative response from the immune system, using system resources and (ironically) increasing the impact of a specific toxin in the body. By deleting these programs, the immune system is free to simply metabolize, ignore, or excrete the toxin.

There are several physical and vibrational techniques for dealing with specific chemical sensitivities. One of the most effective is NAET, an offshoot of acupuncture. With NAET, the person is treated for a specific allergy (normally identified by muscle testing), and for the physical and nonphysical meridians involved. While the patient/client holds a vial containing the allergen, the practitioner uses acupuncture needles in the normal way, or, in some circumstances, can apply NAET techniques from a distance using intention or a QXCI machine. After treatment, the patient/client typically feels an immediate difference. The person avoids the allergen for 25 hours, and will usually check as permanently clear for that allergy. In many case, the client/patient can then resume a normal life, sometimes after years of weakness, illness or fatigue.

EVER-INCREASING TOXICITY

In the past 100 years, awareness of environmental toxins has increased tremendously (even if action is not always taken in a timely manner). In the 19th century, concern about working conditions was confined to a tiny minority of eccentric factory owners and a slightly larger group of union organizers. Certain industries were notorious for their appalling health conditions because of chemical contaminations; many more factory workers had bad health records through a combination of chemical toxins and poor nutrition. The few times factory owners/managers introduced nutritional programs, the health effects of industrial contamination were noticeably reduced. These days there are much more stringent laws regarding environmental pollution, at least in the US, and yet the overall levels of contamination are still quite high enough to affect the health of millions. This is especially true for the more vulnerable parts of our community: children, seniors, and those exposed to industrial processes.

Obviously, the lower the overall intake of toxic chemicals, the better for the person's immune system. At the same time, what a person eats also has a major impact on how such toxins will affect the individual system. Because the basic nutrients are supplied by the daily intake of fats, proteins, carbohydrates, fiber, minerals, and vitamins, overall health is strongly dependent on the quantity and quality of the food we eat. When appropriate nutrients link up to receptor sites, or take their place in the cells, then there is nowhere for the toxins to land. Conversely, when toxic chemicals use up those receptor sites, the correct nutrients are not absorbed. Thus we see that certain toxins not only contaminate the body in themselves, they also displace essential nutrients, thereby causing an additional level of physical, mental, or emotional dysfunction.

Although in theory the Recommended Daily Allowances (RDAs) set by the FDA are enough to keep malnutrition and its associated diseases at bay, the artificial protocols used to set RDAs mean that they are relatively useless as measures of nutritional health. Nutritional research suggests that certain foods and/or supplements can have direct effect on a person's susceptibility to specific toxins.

For instance, for many years we have known that lead is both toxic and wide-spread in the environment: it can be found in petroleum products, paints, glass and ceramic glazes, and many other commonly found chemicals and objects. Lead is stored in the bone marrow, kidneys, liver, and spleen; it has been associated with multiple sclerosis, diabetes, tooth decay, and diminished mental and nervous capacity. These days, even sub-toxic levels of lead contamination are now implicated in ADD, emotional and emotional immaturity, irritability, impulsiveness, and hyperactivity.

Children are noticeably more affected by lead than adults, and poisoning by lead and other metals can lead to nervous system damage and consequent behavioral disorders. Although the brain is ordinarily fairly well protected, young children and babies are more susceptible than adults. Once lead gets into a brain cell, it binds to critical cell parts and cannot be removed. Even at very low levels of lead, this can lead to abnormal brain functioning and disruption of GABA, thereby disturbing the transmission of nerve messages in the brain.

How is nutrition involved in this? Lead is more easily taken up when the body lacks essential elements such as calcium, phosphorus, iron, copper, and magnesium. Increased amounts of sugar, especially lactose, also increase the absorption of lead. Thus a diet rich in minerals but low in sugar will do a great deal to counteract potential lead toxicity. There are similar correlations between other toxins and the level of vitamins, minerals, and other nutrients in a person's body.

Although these days we have stricter limits on toxic contamination in the work place, there is little legal protection from lower levels of contamination arising from the use of everyday objects and chemicals such as cosmetics, solvents, paints, plastics, and foam. Individual industrial processes may have more restrictive limits than previously; however, there is a far larger range of toxic chemicals now being manufactured, in vastly greater quantities. The use of agricultural pesticides alone has increased twelve-fold in the last fifteen years. This means that there is a much higher level of synthetic chemical contamination now than in the heyday of unregulated industrial pollution. If this is the case in a regulated society like the U.S., then how much worse will it be in the rest of the world? We need only remember the chemical disaster at Bhopal, India to see how weaker laws or inattention can poison (or kill) through direct toxic contamination. Bhopal may be far away in terms of miles, yet its toxicity differs from our American circumstances only in level rather than type.

The effect of widespread chemical contamination on humans can be found in the increasing levels of immune and autoimmune dysfunctions. Because the human system is unable to metabolize certain toxins (such at DDT and certain other pesticides, for example), they tend to accumulate in the body. Other manufactured chemicals prevent the uptake of necessary nutrients. Yet another type of contamination is found in chemicals that provoke an allergic reaction from the immune systems of chemically sensitive people. Above all, the increasing range and amount of toxic chemicals creates such work for the immune system that it can no longer protect the body effectively from its designed targets: foreign particles, proteins, and pathogens.

In its efforts to deal with particles that it cannot metabolize, the body has various responses. The immune system can slow down in an effort to handle foreign particles. The body can encapsulate the particles, which can lead to fibrosis and/or allergic reactions. The particles can persuade the target organ to change its own programming, leading to "benign" and cancerous tumors.

To summarize, toxic contaminations can come in through the mouth, lungs, or skin. The impact of a particular toxin depends on the level of genetic or personal sensitivity, combined with nutrition, environmental factors, and the nature of the contamination itself. As well as acute and/or chronic physical poisoning, the major effect of toxicity is to overload the immune system, leading to allergies, lowered immune resistance, and autoimmune diseases.

TYPES OF TOXINS

Of the five types of toxicity mentioned in the introduction, the two that cause the greatest concern in modern society are pesticides and petrochemicals. Both in quantity and quality, these two chemical types have become an increasing burden on everyone's immune system.

Pesticides

We have become so accustomed to dosing ourselves with mosquito repellent that we have mostly forgotten that synthetic pesticides are a recent invention. It is true that the Romans used salt and ashes to sterilize the soil (mainly as a symbolic punishment), and extracts of nicotine and chrysanthemum have been used for several hundred years in both East and West. Pesticide use prior to the last hundred years has occasionally included the use of inorganic compounds, including sulfur, copper, mercury, and arsenic. However, it was only with the development of chemical technologies during World War II that pesticides (and fertilizers) became widely available at an economically viable cost.

The term 'pesticide' means "something that kills pests", of whatever description. Pesticides ("pest killers") are synthetic organic chemicals that are deliberately introduced into the environment in order to selectively poison specific plants (herbicides) insects (insecticides), molds (fungicides), rats/mice (rodenticides), ticks/mites (acaricides), nematocides for worms, termiticides for termites, bactericides to kill bacteria, and so on. Although they may have different targets, many pesticides are essentially similar in composition. Pesticides comprise only 10% of the chemicals used in the U.S., yet they are a particularly prominent group because they are designed to work directly in the environment. Humans are therefore exposed to pesticides and their toxic effects from many different directions: through food, water, soil, and air, in their homes, schools, and places of work.

Within the last 100 years, pesticide production has gone from zero to over *three billion pounds* every year in the US alone. Although 90% of pesticides are used in the agricultural production of food, timber, and fiber (e.g., cotton), another 300 million pounds of anti-fungal ingredients are incorporated into paints, shampoos, dentures, mattresses, paper, wigs, carpets, contact lenses, disposable diapers, and other products. Pesticides are also used in ponds and swimming pools, wood structures, lawns, and golf courses. In fact, the rise in the golf courses alone has added disproportionately to the amount of pesticides now to be found in the water table.

Plants are the most basic food source for both humans and animals: we therefore compete for space, water, and nutrition with a variety of insects, roundworms, plants (called weeds), and plant pathogens. Additional pressure comes from deteriorating weather patterns, increasing desertification, and, most of all, the human population explosion. Increasing competition for food and space means that more and more ingenuity is required to increase crop yields, and modern farmers often see that as requiring ever greater use of pesticides and fertilizers – both of which have toxic effects on land and people as well as pests.

Of the millions of pounds of pesticides sprayed on crops every year, only 1-3% will actually reach their targeted pests, some of which are now becoming pesticide-resistant. (This is similar to what doctors are finding with pathogens that are increasingly resistant to penicillin and other antibiotics.) Thirty years ago, 7% of preharvest crops were damaged by insects and other pests despite the use of 50 million pounds of pesticides. Today, even though 600 million pounds of pesticides are now being used, 13% of preharvest crops are still damaged by insects. Thus, even with a twelve-fold increase in the use of pesticides, there is nearly twice as damage to crops.

Typically, pesticides and fertilizers leave residues just under the skins of grains, fruits, and vegetables. Therefore, washing and peeling vegetables and fruits will help to keep chemical residues from the human system. However, pesticides are regularly detected inside foods as well, and these cannot be easily removed. Furthermore, these contaminated foods are amongst those our children regularly eat at school.

In terms of the effect on humans, pesticides are known to damage the nervous system (both autonomic and central), genitals, heart, lungs, intestines, blood, liver, and kidneys. Many pesticides have been shown to cause cancer and birth defects in animals and humans. Chlorinated compounds have been repeatedly linked to cancer and to changes in the secondary sex characteristics due to their estrogen-like effects. Because pesticides are so widespread, and also able to affect humans at relatively low levels of exposure, we really can't be sure how widespread an impact pesticides have on the human organism. However, evidence is building that suggests that pesticides are becoming a major health challenge.

Health and learning problems have become too prevalent and all-pervasive, making it virtually impossible to pinpoint the factors for individuals whose problems are related to direct or indirect exposure to pesticides. The symptoms often (but not invariably) begin shortly after a major exposure, but chronic long-term illnesses can begin with subtle symptoms, so that cause-and-effect relationships are not readily apparent. Also, it is becoming increasingly clear that specific pesticides can combine with or potentiate with other synthetically produced chemicals in ways that create greatly increased toxicity.

How might a person become exposed to pesticides? In agricultural areas, crops are sprayed or dusted with pesticides without giving notice to the human population. In the U.S., pesticides are regularly sprayed on lawns, athletic fields, trees and shrubs. These outdoor chemicals are then tracked into school buildings, homes, and work areas in amounts that are capable of causing contamination and illness. Of the 44 pesticides known to be used on lawns, 13 have been detected in groundwater, and four are believed to cause cancer. These lawn treatments can be applied by anyone, without precautions.

Aerial spraying of parks and farmlands can potentially cause contamination and illness if the prevailing winds blow towards houses and schools. These chemicals can also enter buildings through ventilation ducts and thus become part of indoor air.

Pesticides are also routinely applied inside home and school buildings to control roaches, ants, fleas, and termites in places like kitchens, bathrooms, walls, and basements. In an enclosed space, the exposure can be 100 times higher than that found outdoors. Although chemicals are usually sprayed in houses and classrooms when they are vacant, sometimes an oily residue is left on furniture and walls; such residues can also cause symptoms as they evaporate and are inhaled, through skin contact, or by ingestion from contact with the fingers.

Therefore, we see that pesticides are ubiquitous, highly and deliberately toxic, and able to affect many physical systems. Children's immune systems tend to be more sensitive than those of adults, yet pesticides are used routinely in schools, parks, and playing fields where children are easily contaminated. We are only now beginning to see just how much impact these common chemicals have on overall health, vitality, and learning abilities.

Petrochemicals

One of the major changes in the industrial landscape is the development of innumerable petrochemicals from fossilized trees: coal, coal tar, and petroleum. Oil-based chemicals are found in the products or production of fuels, foods, paper, textiles, plastics, appliances, adhesives and solvents, paints, computers, pesticides, recording tape... The list is nearly endless. Although we only tend to think of substances like paint or pesticides as chemicals *per se*, in fact there are petrochemical components in virtually every object around us.

As well as finished consumer goods such as computers, toys, and cars, petroleum-based chemicals are part of the manufacturing processes of many more products, whether as raw materials, reactive components, solvents/finishes, or end-products. Without petrochemicals, our society simply could not exist in the form we know now.

When examining the many ways in which chemicals affect the global and personal environment, it's best to start with raw materials. Some minerals and metals are dug directly out of the ground; however, the vast majority of chemicals are created from natural gas and oil. Although preliminary exploration of petrochemicals started in the middle of the 19th century with the invention of coal-tar dyes and similar chemicals, serious development of natural gas and oil technologies began during World War II. As war-related discoveries were taken up by post-War industrialists (and as chemists and inventors were once more free to take up their peace-time occupations), the invention and use of petrochemicals became increasingly widespread both in quality and quantity. In the years between 1950 and 1985, for example, the volume of chemicals produced for industrial uses increased fifty-fold.

The U.S. Department of Commerce classifies the 500 million tons of chemicals produced yearly according to the following eight categories:

1. Industrial inorganic chemicals
2. Industrial organic chemicals
3. Detergents, soaps and toiletries
4. Drugs
5. Paints and finishes
6. Synthetic resins and plastics
7. Agricultural chemicals
8. Miscellaneous chemicals.

As the fourth-largest industry in the U.S., chemical manufacturing is clearly a significant and highly profitable sector of the economy, accounting for over ten percent of the gross national product in the U.S. and therefore trillions of dollars per annum. The positive side of all this chemical manufacturing is the ease, convenience, and pleasure of our modern lifestyle: cars, computers, furniture, books (a much more recent luxury than you would think), synthetic fabrics, pharmaceutical drugs, and the myriad plastic objects with which we are surrounded. The downside of all these petrochemicals is the environmental pollution produced by such widespread industrial activity. Between effluents released routinely into the air and water, the destruction of both species and habitats by ill-regulated and short-sighted industrialists and oil slicks on oceans and beaches arising from accidents such as the *Exxon Valdez*, there are all too many ways that petrochemicals can enter the environment. Pesticides are now being found at all levels of the food chain, while solvents are now showing up in well water. Many chemicals are distributed by air as well, leading to increased levels of involuntary exposure.

At the present time, nearly 90% of carbon-based chemicals (hydrocarbons) are extracted from oil in one form or another. This group includes base chemicals used to manufacture many plastics and solvents, such as benzene, ethylene, propylene, xylene, toluene and butylenes.

Furthermore, many inorganic chemicals such as sulfur and ammonia are produced as byproducts of other processes involving natural gas or oil. This group includes hydrochloric, sulfuric, and other acids, which are used in many manufacturing and industrial processes without ending up in the finished products. Other inorganic chemicals such as halogens are integral ingredients of otherwise organic products such as organochloride pesticides.

Between organic and inorganic processes, petrochemical toxicity is therefore the most widespread type of environmental exposure. Probably the most ubiquitous and harmful petrochemicals are the organic solvents. These are hydrocarbons that are able to dissolve other hydrocarbons, such as oils and waxes. Solvents are used to clean precision parts, dilute glues and paints, clean fabrics, and in various extraction processes.

Solvents are very widely used, both industrially and in the home. The most common types of solvent can be divided into five main types:

1. Alcohols such as ethanol and isopropyl alcohol;

2. Ketones like acetone and methyl ethyl ketone;

3. Aliphatic hydrocarbons such as formaldehyde, ethylene, and acetic acid;

4. Aromatic hydrocarbons like DDT, PCBs, and benzene;

5. Halogenated hydrocarbons such as refrigerants (CFCs), and methylene chloride.

Many solvents are flammable, explosive, corrosive, and/or toxic. Halogenated solvents (those containing iodine, fluorine, bromine, or chlorine) are somewhat less likely to explode or corrode than those without halogens; however, they are still toxic, especially the most commonly used ones, i.e., the chlorinated solvents. There are vast majority of chlorinated solvents are methylene chloride, trichloroethane, trichloroethylene, and tetrachloroethylene. Of the *two billion pounds* or more of chlorinated solvents produced per year in the U.S., possibly 1% gets recycled, with 94% being released into the environment. The remaining 5% are mainly used in plastic products such as food wrap and CFCs.

Focus on recycling, shifts to more benign water-based solvents and breakthroughs in technology mean that the demand for chlorinated solvents is gradually declining. However, because these solvents are such an integral part in such a wide variety of manufactured goods, there will continue to be substantial demand for some time to come. At present, there is very little incentive for the chemical industry to change its dependence on these toxic chemicals.

Unfortunately, by their nature, solvents also have corrosive, toxic effects on the delicate structures of the human body. They can damage the skin, blood, liver, lungs, kidneys, and nervous system. They cause rashes, allergic dermatitis, organ failure, and cancer.

Most solvents evaporate easily; therefore, the most common route of contamination is through the mouth, nose, and lungs. Inhaling these vapors can produce irritation to the lungs and throat, pulmonary edema, arrhthymia, light-headedness, or dizziness, blurred vision, nausea and vomiting, insomnia, nervousness, confusion, unconsciousness, and death. Although acute symptoms often pass when exposure ceases, the lingering effects may only turn up years later in the form of damage to the lungs, liver, and kidneys.

Although most solvent damage occurs through inhalation, people can also become poisoned when groundwater is contaminated through chemical spills, accidents, and leaks. Toxins can also be absorbed through skin contact, and this can cause redness, cracks, and/or scaly patches to develop. Although these symptoms usually heal once the solvent is removed, even a brief contact can lead to allergic reactions and immune system overload.

Paradoxically, solvents that don't cause immediate symptoms are often more dangerous than those that do; at least with direct correlation between exposure and symptoms, the person is alerted to the contamination. Without immediate warning, long-term consequences can come as a very unpleasant surprise when end-organ damage surfaces. Habitual exposure can lead to permanent damage to the lungs, liver, kidneys, and nervous system. Some solvents damage the immune system, others distort the production of blood cells, yet others are implicated in cancer and birth defects. Once solvents are in the blood system, they can pass through the placenta into the fetus and cause lasting damage.

Those who are sensitive to chemical contamination need to find out as much as they can about the solvents in their environment, whether at home, at work, or in public. It can be challenging to find out the composition of proprietary chemicals, but some information is available through the Occupational Safety and Health Administration (OSHA), who can supply Material Safety Data Sheets, which, although sometimes incomplete, still provide useful information for those wishing to safeguard their health.

OSHA will support this type of investigation in the workplace; unfortunately, consumers can find it much more difficult to find out exactly what paints, furniture, and cleaning supplies may contain. Labels are not obliged to list specific solvents as ingredients; in fact, they are often listed as "inert" ingredients, even though the solvents in a given product may well be toxic and/or carcinogenic. Some chemicals aren't even known to be toxic until 20 or 30 years after being released into the environment. The safest course is to eliminate unnecessary chemicals as much as possible from our lives.

CLEARING TOXICITY

With all this cheerful information about the many toxins surrounding us these days, it's good to know that there are ways of addressing both toxicity and chemical sensitivity. When broad-spectrum sensitivity first became known as a medical problem, it seemed as if the only treatment was to isolate sufferers completely – either in the desert or in "clean rooms" that had specially ventilated air, purified water, and a complete absence of paint and furniture finishes. Of course, this inevitably meant the disruption of the person's life, to the detriment of his or her business and family life. Such isolation might last the rest of the person's life, for lack of understanding and treating the underlying causes of chemical sensitivity.

Fortunately, other treatments are now possible. As well as relatively crude drug therapies, allergists are now able to call on allergy clearing treatments to alleviate the strain on the immune system. Vibrational healing modalities are able to address the underlying issues that create a hypersensitive immune system. Treating (or deleting) the cause makes it much easier to deal with the symptoms.

Most people require healing because they have pain or discomfort on a physical level, although long-distance healing is also able to address psychological pain. When something in our body hurts, we tend to lose track of the fact that the physical is just a lower, slower form of vibration. By restoring the correct vibrational frequency, we make it possible for the body to snap back into its ideal energy pattern, and thus support its inherent physical health.

With any kind of vibrational healing, we operate from these three principles:

- Everything is energy.

- Everything and everyone has a frequency.

- Those frequencies that are out of balance with our natural harmony can be identified and removed.

We live at the threshold of a universal recognition that the human being is not mere matter but a potent, energetic field of consciousness. Modalities of the past millennium are quickly giving way to breakthrough technologies where we heal ourselves at the level of all true healing, which is spirit. In spirit, there is neither time nor place. It is an extraordinary gift to be anywhere in the world and be able to address an energetic imbalance, and wake up the next morning feeling great and ready for a new day.

From an energetic standpoint, the human body, when weakened or shifted from equilibrium, oscillates at a lower and less harmonious frequency. This abnormal frequency reflects a general state of cellular energetic imbalance within the physical body. When a weakened individual is unable to shift his/her energetic mode to the needed frequency, a certain amount of subtle energetic help may be needed to allow the immune system to defend the body effectively. If this same individual is supplied with a dose of the needed energetic frequency, it allows the cellular bioenergetic system to resonate in the proper vibrational mode, thereby throwing off the toxicities of the illness. This frequency-specific subtle energy boost allows the physical body and associated bioenergy systems to return to a new level of homeostasis.

If the frequency match is correct and the needed energy is supplied to the patient, healing occurs quickly and easily. Frequently, the final resolution of illness is preceded by an exacerbation of symptoms known as a "healing crisis". This type of crisis is an indication of the physical body resonating at the needed energy frequency, causing the transient intensification of the symptoms of toxic release. Only an exact frequency match will cause a healing because, by the principle of resonance, biological systems only accept certain resonant frequencies that "match" the inherent coding and allow the system to move toward a new level of energetic organization and function.

An analogy for this process can be found in computers. We know that we can only produce output from what the computer already has in it by way of programs, information, and so on. When a computer is wired correctly, contains the right programs for a specific task, and is switched on, then it can perform its tasks with speed and efficiency.

One of the more serious problems for computers is the existence of computer viruses. These are "mini-programs" designed to interrupt the normal functioning of a computer. If there is a virus in your system, it will cause the computer to crash, run a program you don't want, and/or use up system resources in evading the virus. Most computers have the equivalent of an immune system in the form of viral scanning programs such as McAfee or Norton. When the viral scanning program comes across codes that it doesn't recognize, it has the choice of allowing the virus or isolating and destroying the virus. When a virus is isolated and destroyed, the computer is able to return to its normal efficiency. When toxins and allergens are identified and dissolved, the human body is able to spring back to its full level of health with speed and efficiency. The result for the human being is a rapid increase in vitality, emotional balance, and physical strength.

In order to identify and destroy computer viruses, the viral scanning program requires the "signature" of the virus, which it then compares with an internal list to discover if the virus's coding is allowable or not. If the viral scanning program cannot identify the virus, it will not be able to take appropriate action. In the same way, the human immune system has to know whether a particular chemical or pathogen is "allowed" or whether it needs to quarantine and destroy that substance. One of the difficulties with all the modern chemicals and toxins is that they are more difficult for the immune system to identify. The effect on human health is to "stall" the immune system, glands, and/or other organs. The effects normally surface in the person's weakest organ or meridian, causing it to slow or crash.

So we can see that toxins and disease can have the same effect on the human body as computer viruses can have in a computer. The good news is that, like a computer, the body can quickly and easily bounce back from contamination, once the toxin has been identified. Obviously a part of the healing can rest in simply removing the toxin or allergen from the environment, yet at times this is neither practical nor desirable. The "signature" of the toxin must also be removed for the immune system to register which conditions to allow and which to eliminate, and this can be done vibrationally through programs like NAET. In fact, the genius of NAET lies in the identification and release of specific toxins, and a treatment very frequently leads to the immediate release of symptoms and rapid restoration of physical health and vitality as the immune system is enabled to resume its proper functioning.

VIBRATIONAL HEALING

The brilliant German physician Samuel Hahnemann (1755-1843) developed a system of treatment based on the unique principle of "like cures like" – that is, he treated diseases with medicines known to reproduce the symptoms of the disease. This principle led directly to homeopathy and other vibrational modalities. In homeopathy, a remedy is chosen for its ability to stimulate and rebalance the physical body through supplying the needed frequency of subtle energy. If the remedy's frequency matches the patient's illness state, a transfer of energy will allow the patient's bioenergetic system to assimilate the needed energy, thus releasing the toxic energy pattern and moving the body to a new equilibrium point of health.

Our long-distance healing uses the same principle to affect the individual's bioenergetic frequency. Using a photograph to provide an energy interference pattern, subtle energy imbalances can be identified and specific balancing can be imprinted on the individual's energy field. Once the subtle energy blockages that impede a person's natural ability to keep in top condition are removed, the person normally experiences an upsurge of physical energy as well as the clearing of the original symptoms. This can take place on the physical, mental, emotional, and spiritual levels. As negative frequencies are removed from the energetic field, a person is able to express his or her life more fully and completely. Obviously, this means different things to different people – increased vitality for one, more flexibility for another, possibly more creativity for a third. Rather than being caught up in the pain of the past and the fear of the future, most people also experience a greater sense of living Here and Now, an ability to stay calm and balanced, and better focus on their work, family or other concerns.

A wide variety of toxic sensitivities can be addressed by vibrational healing techniques, especially Nambudrapad's Allergy Elimination Technique (NAET), a modality that specifically addresses allergic reactions. NAET is an offshoot of acupuncture. Dr. Devi Nambudrapad, an acupuncturist based in Los Angeles, discovered that when she applied existing acupuncture techniques for the alleviation of allergic symptoms *while the patient was holding the allergen*, s/he would be cleared of that allergic reaction. If the patient avoids exposure to that allergen for 25–30 hours afterwards, s/he will, in most cases, be permanently free of that allergy. Occasionally a second treatment will be required for the allergen or toxin, but for most people one treatment is sufficient to clear toxins that they have suffered from all their lives. In effect, the NAET treatment has removed a computer virus from the person's system, allowing it to function efficiently again.

Although normally performed in person, certain practitioners have also found NAET to be effective when carried out using long-distance techniques such as the QXCI healing program. (QXCI is a computer program that operates in subspace. It is capable of reading a person's energetic signature and rectifying unbalanced conditions both in person and across any distance, so long as the practitioner provides an appropriate link to the patient/client.) The vibrational approach to NAET is beneficial as clients need not come to a specific location for treatment. In fact, treatment frequently takes place at night, so that the patient can relax at home and simply avoid the relevant foods or other substances during the next day. Distance healing also enables the practitioner to treat more people than those limited to office hours.

Unlike physical healing techniques that rely on direct contact, vibrational healing operates in the energy fields, where there is neither time nor space. There are many more vibrational modalities besides NAET or QXCI. (In fact, the latest QXCI program, called SCIO, offers 240 modalities, including Bach flower remedies, chiropractic, homeopathy, and direct energetic application of herbs and minerals.) As well as making treatment times and locations more flexible, vibrational healing can be used to address other levels of the person than the strictly physical. The emotional body, mental body, causal body, and other energy bodies are as important to the human energy structure as the physical body with its physical symptoms. Treating or releasing toxins from other energy levels is important in itself, and can be a vital part of healing the physical organism.

As Einstein said, problems cannot be solved at the level of manifestation; you need to find a solution at a higher level. Instead of the slow, sometimes painful process of detoxification and other treatments that focus solely on the physical body, vibrational healing operates on the level of the person's essential energy patterns. Once these are restored, it is much easier to bring the physical symptoms back into balance.

Because *everything* is vibration, vibrational remedies are capable of resetting any type of frequency distortion. Once the energy pattern is restored, it is relatively easy to restore the physical health as well. In fact, the overall frequency or "center of gravity" determines what level of healing a person requires. Those at a lower frequency may well need physical measures such as surgery or drugs. Those of medium frequency usually respond well to homeopathy and acupuncture. At higher frequencies, 'pure' vibrational techniques are enough to restore the pattern of health.

What are the benefits here? Vibrational healing offers a very rapid and effective way of resetting the body's natural level of health. In contrast to traditional or allopathic medicine, vibrational healing offers:

- The ability to diagnose and clear mysterious or "unknown" conditions.

- Rapid and complete relief of physical and nonphysical symptoms.

- Speedier healing times than generally experienced with radiation, chemo-therapy or surgery.

- Complete absence of unfortunate side-effects from drugs or misdiagnosis.

- Permanent release from specific allergic and toxic conditions.

The body has a built-in pattern of health, part of the divine design for each individual's life. When we release anything that distorts that pattern, and supply the proper nutrients, water, rest, and exercise, then the body will rapidly restore its own equilibrium. The innate body intelligence knows exactly where the person is, how they got there, and how to get them out again into full health. As healers, we only need to tap into that intelligence to assist our patients/clients to the living experience of their own homeostatic balance once more.

TOXINS LIST

In this section you will find a list of toxins, each with symptoms and sources.

ACRYLIC

Acrylic is a synthetic plastic resin derived from acroleic acids and is used in a wide range of industrial, commercial, and household products.

Symptoms

1. Corrosion of eyes, skin, respir. system
1. Sore throat
1. Pulmonary edema
1. Diarrhea
1. Headache
1. Lightheadedness
1. Irritation of skin, redness/swelling
1. Kidney damage
1. Changes to memory/concentration
1. May damage the developing fetus
1. Weakness, fatigue
1. Cough
1. Burning sensation
1. Abdominal cramps
1. Reproductive toxicity

16. Dental odors
17. Shortness of breath
18. Skin sensitivity
19. Unconsciousness
20. Dizziness
21. Irritation and watering of eyes
22. Dermatitis
23. Possible damage to the nervous system
24. Abnormal liver or kidney function
25. Nausea, vomiting
26. Diarrhea
27. Prolonged menstrual cycles
28. Gastrointestinal irritation
29. Depression
30. Can cause cancer

Sources

1. Clothing, yarn fibers, sanitary napkins
1. Brushes
1. Paints and glazes, home maintenance
1. Plastic key rings, dispensers, tags
1. Lucite, Plexiglas, acrylic jewelry
1. Hot tubs, bathtubs, showers
1. Aquariums
1. Pet care: flea and tick control
1. Light boxes, photo frames
1. Dentures, food prep, household cleaners

11. Fake nails, makeup, soap, hairspray
12. Furniture with acrylic finish
13. Resurfacing asphalt, concrete
14. Linoleum, floor finishes, floor wax
15. Tires and auto products
16. Carpeting
17. Specialty Upholstery
18. Synthetic blankets
19. Roofing materials
20. PVC pipes

ALUMINUM

A naturally occurring element, aluminum is a medium-hard silvery metal often used in the aerospace industry and for many household objects. In general, aluminum is ingested, although it is sometimes absorbed through the skin. Aluminum has been implicated in Alzheimer's.

Symptoms

1. Dyspepsia
1. Ulcers
1. Heartburn
1. Colitis
1. Gastric hyperactivity
1. Dry skin and mucus membranes
1. Profound debility, heaviness, numbness
1. Burning in head with vertigo
1. Aversion to meat, potatoes disagree
1. Premature aging
11. Flatulence
12. Headaches
13. Digestive disturbances
14. Nephritic and hepatic disorders
15. Nervous symptoms
16. Paralysis
17. Head colds and eructation
18. Throbbing headache with constipation
19. Colic, similar to painter's colic
20. Rigidity in blood vessels

Sources

1. Cookware and utensils
1. Canned foods
1. Drinking water (some types)
1. Children's aspirin
1. Bleached white flours
1. Skin moisturizers
1. Salt
1. Salts for water softeners
1. Shower doors
1. Beer and soft drink cans
1. Automobile parts
1. Window frames
13. Baking powder
14. Aluminum foil
15. Bases for false teeth
16. Antacids
17. Detergents and soaps
18. Deodorants, even "aluminum free"
19. Walkers
20. Lipsticks
21. Bathroom supports
22. Aluminum paints
23. Desiccants
24. Deck chairs

ALUMINUM FLUORIDE

Aluminum fluoride is an inorganic compound mainly ingested through the mouth by drinking water that has been contaminated.

Symptoms

1. Can cause cancer
1. Mottling of the teeth
1. Kidney/bladder disorders
1. Vomiting
1. Excessive thirst
1. Arthritis
1. Nervousness
1. Mouth ulcers
1. Bronchitis
1. Brittle nails
1. Numbness
1. Skin problems
1. Allergies
1. Heart disease
1. Advances aging

16. Wrinkled skin
17. Prickly sensation in muscles
18. Constipation
19. Itching after bathing
20. Headaches
21. Gum diseases
22. Hair loss
23. Vision problems
24. Weakening of the immune system
25. Sinus problems
26. Stomach disorders
27. Mutagenic
28. Dental deformities
29. Birth defects
30. Leads to aluminum deposits in bones

Sources

1. Toothpaste

2. City drinking water supplies

ANTIMONY

This is a naturally occurring element that is used in many industrial processes. It can get into the system through ingestion, by skin contact, or through the dust of mining and/or refining. Contamination can sometimes resemble arsenical poisoning.

Symptoms

1. Mucus membrane irritation
1. Irritated lining of alimentary tract
1. Cardiac and arterial depression
1. Poisoning to cardiac muscle
1. Pigmented pustules
1. GI tract congestion/edema
1. Weakness
1. Bleeding gums
1. Laryngitis
1. Itching skin pustules

11. Rashes
12. Watery stools
13. Dehydration
14. Hepatic damage
15. Physical collapse
16. Headaches
17. Anemia
18. Conjunctivitis
19. Unexplained weight loss
20. Pre-cancerous and cancerous tumors
21. Sciatic Pain

Sources

1. Printing type
1. Munitions
1. Safety matches
1. Pewter utensils
1. Foil
1. Textiles
1. Emetics and vermifuges

8. Storage batteries
9. Paint pigments
10. Vulcanized red rubber
11. Metallic alloys
12. Pharmaceuticals
13. Ant paste
14. Ore refining dust and fumes

ARSENIC

Arsenic is a naturally-occurring element that is most often found in manufactured form as a white powder. In the past, arsenic was widely used as a rat poison, in medicines used to thin the blood, in cosmetics, and as an ingredient in wallpaper glue.

Symptoms

1. Abdominal pain
1. Jaundice
1. Liver inflammation/degeneration
1. Exfoliate erythroderma
1. Sore throats (esp. in children)
1. Peripheral neuropathy
1. Encephalopathy
1. Peripheral vascular disease
1. Myocardial infarctions
1. Hepatic vasculature
1. Hypertension, nervousness
1. Headache
1. Drowsiness, fatigue
1. Confusion, cognitive impairment
1. Seizures, nervous exhaustion
1. Hyperkeratosis of the palms of the hands
1. Sweet metallic taste
1. Stomach toxicity

19. Psychological disturbances
20. Lung, skin, throat, bladder cancer
21. Tumors to internal organs
22. Systolic blood pressure changes
23. Raynaud's disease (vasoconstriction)
24. Renal tubular dysfunction
25. Inhibited respiration
26. Urinary dysfunction
27. Spinal subluxations, backaches
28. Facial edema with red discoloration
29. Pigmented scars, neck, armpits, nipples
30. Pigmented pustules in areas of sweat
31. Burning eyes, throat, chest, tonsils
32. Hair loss, brittle nails
33. Anemia, anorexia
34. Throat constriction
35. Tremors
36. Weakness, listlessness

Sources

1. Tobacco smoke
1. Weed killers
1. Pesticides
1. Drinking water
1. Wine substitutes
1. Mining and ore-refining

7. Dental compounds for root canals
8. Industrial effluents
9. Manufacturing of glass
10. Coal smoke
11. Insecticides
12. Medicines

ASBESTOS

ASBESTOS is a generic term for the fibrous forms of several mineral silicates. These occur naturally in seams or veins, generally between about 1 and 20 millimeters (mm) in width in many igneous or metamorphic rocks, and belong to one of two large groups of rock forming minerals: the serpentines and the amphiboles. Although the United States banned the use of asbestos in homes and many consumer products, other countries – including Canada – continue to produce the toxic material.

A long-term danger to using feminine hygiene sprays on a regular basis is that most such deodorants contain talc, which can be contaminated with asbestos. Eye shadow, powdered blush, and face powder also contain talc. Urban air frequently contains sprayed asbestos fireproofing used in buildings. In addition, 24 out of 28 lungs were examined were found to contain significant number of asbestos fibers.

Symptoms

1. Can cause cancers, esp. lung, larynx, gall bladder upper throat, kidney, esophagus

1. Pleurisy

1. Cyanosis

1. Possible cause of stomach cancer

5. Causes asbestosis: shortness of breath, chronic cough, abnormal lung sounds

6. Clubbing to fingers and toes

7. Failure of right side of the heart

8. Possible genetic link

9. Nail abnormalities

Sources

1. Hair dryers

1. Drier fan belt

1. Ironing board covers, stove top pads

1. Insulation and fireproofing

1. Talc and baby powder

1. Asbestos cement pipes

1. Vinyl floor tile and sheet flooring

1. Roofing shingles

1. Wallboard and joint compound

1. Asbestos ceiling and floor tiles

1. Cement

1. Acoustical materials

13. Asbestos gloves

14. Corrugated building facings/siding

15. Pre-1970 clutch and brake linings

16. High-voltage electrical cords

17. Roofing paper or felt

18. Flexible duct connectors

19. Asbestos tape

20. Furnace cement

21. Roofing materials

22. Pipe coverings/insulation

23. Gaskets

24. Appliance and wiring insulation

ASPARTAME

A sweetener discovered by accident in 1965, aspartame is an odorless white powder soluble in water and alcohol, not fats or oils. Scientists are concerned about its excessive use as an ingredient in many processed foods because aspartame contains an amino acid called aspartate that is known to stimulate the brain. This over-stimulation can damage the brain, possibly leading to neurological diseases. Unborn children are particularly as risk, as aspartate may cross the placenta to affect brain development.

Symptoms

1. Severe itching
1. Behavioral changes
1. Diarrhea
1. Dizziness, memory loss, brain fog
1. Slurred speech, burning tongue
1. Hyperactivity, aggression
1. Seizures and convulsions
1. Hives
1. Swollen lips, mouth, tongue and throat
1. Birth and brain defects
1. Hopelessness, depression, suicide
1. Nightmares, sleeplessness
1. Chronic fatigue, lupus
1. Phobias, allergic reactions, asthma
1. Excessive hunger or thirst, craving sweets
1. Parkinson's disease, MS or ALS
1. Lost balance, uncontrolled movements
1. Lymphoma
1. Bell's palsy

20. Multiple chemical sensitivities
21. Nervousness, anxiety, panic attacks
22. Aches and pains, headaches, migraines
23. Brain tumors
24. Rapid heart beat, tachycardia
25. Impotency and sexual problems
26. Blood sugar control problems
27. Edema
28. Tingling legs or feet
29. Loss of sense of taste
30. Acne or facial pain, face flushing
31. Fibromyalgia
32. Phobias, anxiety
33. Arthritis
34. Peripheral neuropathy
35. Weight gain (can be extreme)
36. Abdominal pain, menstrual problems
37. Susceptibility to infection
38. Interstitial cystitis (blood in urine, pain)

Sources

1. Coca Cola and other sodas, diet sodas
1. Twin Lab products (select items)
1. Gum or breath mints
1. Some cereals
1. Sugar-free sweeteners
1. Lite beer
1. Non-prescription pharmaceuticals

8. Ready-mixed beverages
9. Sugar-free chocolate
10. Processed foods and drinks
11. Spices, natural flavorings
12. Toothpaste
13. MSG
14. Soy protein, gravies, yeast extract

BENZENE

Benzene is a colorless, highly flammable liquid with a characteristic odor. It tends to target the liver and also accumulate in the thyroid.

Symptoms

1. Dizziness
1. Headache
1. Nausea
1. Ventricular arrhythmia
1. Convulsions
1. Leukemia
7. Weakness
8. Euphoria
9. Vomiting
10. Paralysis
11. Aplastic anemia
12. Weakens immune system, bone marrow

Sources

1. Hydrocarbons
1. Phenolics such as toluene, xylene
1. Charcoal-broiled and/or smoked foods
1. Fuel additive
1. Artificially flavored foods, esp. sweets
1. Bottled water and fruit juice
1. Cold cereals, including health brands
1. Hand creams moisturizers
1. Vaseline products, chap stick
1. Personal lubricants
1. Cattle and poultry feeds
1. Airplane glue
1. Cigarette and coal smoke
1. Solvents for wax, resins, rubber
15. Cooking oil, shortening
16. Toothpaste, including health brands
17. Ice cream and frozen yogurt
18. Chewing gum
19. Vitamins and health supplements
20. Tea tree oil products (ex. Thursday Plan.)
21. Flavored pet foods (cats and dogs)
22. Bird food made into cakes
23. Dyes
24. Store bought flavors
25. Grilled foods
26. Hot dogs and lunch meats
27. Beer

BERYLLIUM

Beryllium is an element found in nature in the form of an extremely hard and lightweight metal. It's a non-magnetic electrical conductor; chronic exposure to breathing beryllium dust or fumes may cause serious lung diseases amongst industrial workers. Domestically, 70% of beryllium exposure comes from drinking water, and 30% from food sources.

Symptoms

1. Unexplained cough
1. Chronic pneumonia or bronchitis
1. Shortness of breath with activity
1. Night sweats
1. Fatigue
1. Fever
1. Skin disease, rash, wart-like bumps

8. Poor wound healing
9. Higher risk of lung cancer
10. Small lung scars on chest x-ray
11. Increased calcium in urine
12. General weakness or debility
13. Granuloma scars in lung or skin
14. Weight loss, loss of appetite

Sources

1. Jet brake pads
1. Aerospace components
1. Ignition modules
1. Rocket covers
1. X-ray windows
1. Transistors
1. Heat shields
1. Pre-1951 fluorescent lamps/tubes
1. Dental alloys
1. Coal and fuel oil
1. Cattle and poultry feeds

12. Copper and aluminum alloys
13. Semi-conductor chips
14. Jet engine blades
15. Nuclear reactors and weapons
16. Chemistry and metallurgy
17. Metallic ores
18. Scrap metals
19. Golf clubs, bicycle frames
20. Tobacco smoke
21. Dust from work clothes

BISMUTH

Although the element bismuth is rarely used in industry, its frequent therapeutic uses can give rise to drug poisoning. The chief sources are colloidal bismuth preparations used in the treatment of syphilis. American bismuth is obtained as a by-product in the refining of lead and copper.

Symptoms

1. Excessive salivation
1. Bloody diarrhea
1. Rheumatic pain
1. Renal and liver damage
1. Gingivitis
1. Musculoskeletal abnormalities
1. Neurosis, psychosis
1. Alzheimer's, sometimes sudden onset
1. Blackish line around neck of tooth/gums
1. Protein in the urine, toxic nephrosis

11. Dermatitis
12. Indigestion
13. Respiratory weakness
14. Pyorrhea, possibly causing loss of teeth
15. Hyproadrenalism
16. Decreased appetite
17. Foul breath
18. Conjunctival hemorrhage
19. Temporary encephalopathy/seizures
20. Vesicular erythroderma (skin)

Sources

1. Jet brake pads
1. Aerospace components
1. Ignition modules
1. Rocket covers
1. X-ray windows
1. Transistors
1. Heat shields
1. Pre-1951 fluorescent lamps/tubes
1. Dental alloys
1. Coal and fuel oil
1. Cattle and poultry feeds

12. Copper and aluminum alloys
13. Semi-conductor chips
14. Jet engine blades
15. Nuclear reactors and weapons
16. Chemistry and metallurgy
17. Metallic ores
18. Scrap metals
19. Golf clubs, bicycle frames
20. Tobacco smoke
21. Dust from work clothes

Medical uses

1. Syphilis treatment
1. Astringent action in treating diarrhea
1. Additives in working steel and aluminum
1. Pearl white paint pigment
1. Used in liquid metal fission reactors

6. Antacid action for indigestion
7. Protecting mucus membranes
8. Dental amalgams
9. Used to manufacture pharmaceuticals
10. Treating gastric and duodenal ulcers

CADMIUM

Cadmium is an element found in nature. It is used in the manufacture of many items such as paints and pigments, fertilizers, tobacco, and foodstuffs.

Symptoms

1. Disrupts absorption of other minerals
2. Effect enzyme functions
3. Pneumonitis
4. Vomiting
5. Stomach and bowel irritation
6. Loss of calcium in bones
7. Prostration, exhaustion and fatigue
8. Insomnia with early waking
9. Hypertension
10. Kidney damage
11. Headache
12. Anemia
13. Degeneration of liver and heart
14. Leg pain
15. Parasites and roundworms
16. High blood pressure
17. Glaucoma
18. Chronic indigestion
19. Alzheimer's
20. Breast lumps through accumulation
21. Cardiovascular disease
22. Strokes
23. Chronic rhinitis, loss of sense of smell
24. Dryness of pharynx
25. Proteinuria
26. Tiredness
27. Pulmonary emphysema
28. Liver and kidney stones
29. Toxic hepatitis, liver cirrhosis
30. Cough
31. Diarrhea

Sources

1. Melting alloys
2. Pigments
3. Tobacco leaves and smoke
4. Paints and pigments
5. Contaminated drinking water
6. Glazed crockery
7. Dairy products
8. Fertilizers
9. Sewage sludge
10. Batteries
11. Dental partials and dentures, gold fillings
12. Welding
13. Oxide dusts
14. Galvanized pipes
15. Grains
16. Meats and fish
17. Auto exhaust
18. Acid foods: fruit juices, wine, lemonade

CAMPHOR

Camphor is an aromatic solvent with a very distinctive smell. In the past, it was most often found in moth-proofing compounds and smelling salts!

Symptoms

1. Nausea and vomiting
2. Confusion
3. Vertigo and dizziness
4. Restlessness
5. Hallucinations
6. Jerky movements
7. Respiratory failure
8. Convulsions (stimulating cerebral cortex)
9. Visual disturbances
10. Hepatic derangement
11. Kidney lesions
12. Changes in GI tract, kidneys and brain
13. Excessive thirst
14. Muscle spasms
15. Slow respiration
16. Dilation of the pupils
17. Breath and urine smell of camphor
18. Feeling of warmth
19. Headaches
20. Excitement
21. Delirium
22. Tremors
23. Depression
24. Noises in the ear
25. Gastric distress
26. Urinary retention
27. Hemorrhages
28. Insomnia
29. Burning in mouth and throat
30. Irrational behavior
31. Rapid pulse
32. Rigidity
33. Cold perspiration
34. Reflex spasm of the glottis

Sources

1. Nail enamel
2. Hobby/craft materials
3. Shaving cream
4. Cosmetics
5. Lotions
6. Respiratory aid and stimulant

CARBON MONOXIDE

A colorless asphyxiant gas, carbon monoxide is a constituent of engine exhaust and other fumes; one of the oldest known toxins, it is flammable and possibly explosive.

Symptoms

1. Nausea
2. Headaches
3. Dizziness
4. Unconsciousness and sometimes death
5. Persistent asthma
6. Memory and concentration problems
7. Amblyopia
8. Diplopia
9. Heart palpitations
10. Hypoxia
11. Depression
12. Chronic fatigue
13. Chest pain
14. Behavioral changes
15. Mood changes
16. Hallucinations
17. Choroidal congestion
18. Tiredness
19. Mental dullness
20. Cell death in the heart and blood vessels

Sources

1. Electric furnaces
2. Gas manufacturing plants
3. Charcoal ovens
4. Kilns
5. Commercial laundries
6. Garages
7. Kitchen stoves and ovens
8. Train and bus exhaust
9. Blast furnaces
10. Oil distilleries
11. Refuse plants
12. Coal mines
13. Commercial tailoring irons
14. Industrial and house fires
15. Gas fires and furnaces
16. Auto exhaust

CARBON TETRACHLORIDE

First used in 1839, carbon tetrachloride is a widespread air-borne toxin, as it takes nearly 50 years to break down in the atmosphere. People with pre-existing hepatic damage (e.g., those with alcoholism, diabetes, renal disease, hypertension, cardiac decompensation) are particularly susceptible. As well as being widely used in cleaning products, carbon tet also gets into drinking water from polyvinyl chloride (PVC) water supply pipes. Although it can be removed by filters or boiling, the later simply releases carbon tetrachloride into the air.

Symptoms

1. Disturbance of protein synthesis
2. Confusion
3. Rise in transaminases and serum iron
4. Gastrointestinal disturbances
5. Enlarged, tender liver
6. Liver cell necroses, fatty accumulation
7. Anorexia
8. Gastroduodenal ulcers
9. Heart arrhythmia
10. Leukocytes and erythrocytes in urine
11. Cough with blood-tinged mucus
12. Allergic eczema
13. Convulsions/coma
14. Elevated LDH,
15. Skin contact blistering or ulceration
16. Jaundice
17. Damage to liver, kidneys, lungs, CNS
18. Feelings of drunkenness
19. Fall in prothrombin
20. Giddiness, visual disturbances
21. Aplastic anemia
22. Loss of coordination
23. Birth defects
24. Tiredness or drowsiness
25. Weight loss
26. Dizziness/vertigo
27. Harmful changes in the blood
28. Anxiety

Sources

1. Paint
2. Cleaning liquids
3. Used to degrease metal parts
4. Cleaning agent in dry-cleaning, textiles
5. Disinfectants
6. Contaminated drinking water
7. Pesticide fumigants on grain
8. Rubber products
9. Varnish
10. Solvent for fats, asphalt, rubber, gums
11. Chemical in fire extinguishers
12. Commercial spot removers
13. Fluorocarbon propellant in aerosols
14. Chlorinated paraffin wax

CESIUM

Cesium was the first element to be discovered using a spectroscope; its name, the Latin for "sky blue", refers to the characteristic blue spectral lines of this element. Because cesium binds strongly to soils, plant uptake is by direct absorption into the leaves rather than through the roots. Its principle use is in development research on ion propulsion and thermionic, turboelectric and electrical power generation. Cesium is also used in medical radiation and biological research.

Symptoms

1. Depression
2. Destruction of bone marrow
3. Accumulates in tissues and brain
4. Hyper-irritability

Sources

1. Drinking beverages from plastic bottles
2. Nuclear isotopes used in medicine
3. Meat, milk and grains
4. Infrared signaling lamps, photophones
5. Manufacturing optical crystals
6. Cesium beam atomic clocks
7. Nuclear weapons testing
8. Irradiation of US mail to clear anthrax
9. Photoelectric cells
10. Vacuum tubes
11. Biological research

CHLORINE

A naturally occurring element, chorine is noted for the many ways it can combine to form chemical compounds such as chlorides and chlorates. These days, it is widely used as a disinfectant in swimming pools, town water, and cleaning fluids.

Symptoms

1. Nausea and vomiting
2. Blisters
3. Headaches
4. Sneezing
5. Hoarseness or loss of voice
6. Pneumonitis
7. Dizziness
8. Changes in sensitivity to light
9. Bleaching of hair
10. Heart palpitations
11. Anxiety
12. Pulmonary edema
13. Red and watery eyes
14. Coughing
15. Chest pain
16. Choking
17. Dermatitis
18. Chemical conjunctivitis
19. Fatigue
20. Eye and skin burns

Sources

1. School chemistry experiments
2. Cleaning agents
3. Clorox
4. Swimming pools
5. Yard granules
6. Some laundry products

COBALT

Cobalt is an element that occurs in nature; it is most commonly used as a pigment, in producing metals and glass, to make pharmaceutical drugs, and in fertilizers. Radioactive forms such as Cobalt 60 are used in medical radiation.

Symptoms

1. Nausea
2. Mild collapse
3. Myxedema
4. Abdominal colic
5. Piercing pains in back and chest
6. Nerve deafness
7. Polcythemia
8. Dermatitis
9. Low blood pressure
10. Hypothyroidism
11. Damage to the myelin sheathes
12. Anemia
13. Slow growth rate
14. Vomiting
15. Goiter (swollen thyroid)
16. Generalized pain
17. Severe dyspnea
18. Shortness of breath
19. Hypotension
20. Convulsions
21. Pericardial effusion
22. Metabolic acidosis
23. Itching
24. Nerve damage
25. Fatigue
26. Poor circulation

Sources

1. Cobalt 60 in irradiated plastics
2. Tool steels and magnetic steels
3. Glass-metal sealing alloys
4. Anchoring dentures to neighboring teeth
5. Fertilizers for human and animal foods
6. Toothpaste dyes
7. Humidity indicator for desiccants
8. Aircraft turbine parts
9. Glass colorants
10. Bone replacements
11. Surgical implants
12. Pharmaceuticals
13. Paint, ink and other pigments
14. Undercoat for vitreous enamels

CRESOL

Also called methyl phenol or cresylic acid, this is obtained from the distillation of coal tar (and is therefore one of the many petrochemicals). The crude material is a brownish-yellow liquid that solidifies at 52°F. Traditionally, phenol was used in paints and varnishes; it is still a commonly found solvent with many industrial uses.

Symptoms

1. Skin anesthesia, leading to more toxicity
2. Giddiness
3. Vomiting
4. Headache
5. Tinnitus
6. Insomnia
7. Damage to kidneys
8. Muscle contractions
9. Profuse sweating
10. Abdominal pain
11. Diarrhea
12. Damage to central nervous system
13. Intense thirst
14. Pulmonary edema
15. Pneumonia
16. Jaundice

Sources

1. Plastics
2. Ore flotation
3. Strong antiseptics such as Lysol
4. Photographic developers
5. Paints and varnishes
6. Paint and varnish removers
7. Pharmaceuticals
8. Refining petroleum
9. Disinfectants
10. Fumigants
11. Production of herbicides
12. Printing inks and solvents
13. Preservatives in leather, glue, perfume
14. Thymol, ingredient in cold/cough syrups

DIAZINON

Diazinon is an organophosphate, which can be absorbed by inhalation, ingestion, and skin penetration, and affect the nervous system. Derived from nerve gas agents developed during World War II, it is used as an organic insecticide and has many other agricultural, commercial, and household uses.

Acute symptoms

1. Nausea
2. Headache
3. Tearing
4. Drowsiness
5. Anxiety
6. Reproductive difficulties
7. Muscle twitching
8. Lung congestion
9. Seizures (more common in children)
10. Dizziness
11. Salivation
12. Sweating
13. Agitation
14. Flu-like symptoms
15. Abnormal heart rate
16. Pinpoint pupils
17. Cardiac arrest
18. Allergic skin reactions

Chronic symptoms

1. Headaches
2. Lethargy
3. Inability to concentrate
4. Lowered intelligence test scores
5. Irritability
6. Brain cancer in children
7. Muscle weakness
8. Short term memory loss
9. Confusion
10. Depression
11. Xeno-estrogen effects, inc. colon cancer
12. Non-Hodgkin's lymphoma

Sources

1. Pesticides: Ortho, Spectracide, Real-Kill
2. Lawn sprays
3. Ant and roach killers
4. Insecticides

DIETHYLENE GLYCOL

This is an alcohol-like solvent, frequently found in mechanical systems such as cars and industrial machinery.

Symptoms

1. Nausea and vomiting
2. Abdominal pain
3. Pulmonary edema
4. Distended veins
5. Enlarged/toxic liver
6. Back pain referred to kidneys
7. Renal failure
8. Brain damage
9. Hypotension
10. Hypoglycemia
11. Peripheral nervous disturbances
12. Giddiness
13. Anorexia
14. Diarrhea
15. Headaches
16. Pericardial hemorrhage
17. Enlarged or necrotic kidneys
18. Stomach/intestinal congestion
19. Stomach/intestinal bleeding
20. Eye, skin and respiratory irritations
21. Tachycardia
22. Muscle tenderness
23. Forgetfulness
24. Anemia
25. Sleeplessness
26. Bulimia

Sources

1. Antifreeze coolant
2. Brake fluid
3. Automobile radiators
4. Solvents and lubricants
5. Home maintenance
6. Joint compound
7. Starching collars
8. Filling agents for hydraulic systems

DIOXIN

Otherwise known as Agent Orange, dioxin is thought to be one of the most toxic chemicals made by man. A mutagenic agent, it became notorious towards the end of the Vietnam War for the contact and systemic damages to soldiers and their subsequent children. Very low doses are suspected to cause human illness. It is an unavoidable by-product of the manufacture of certain herbicides and preservatives. There are no known beneficial uses of dioxin.

Symptoms

1. Liver injury
2. Changes to central nervous system
3. Environment for intestinal flukes
4. Damage to intestines, diverticuli
5. Tissue damage
6. Peripheral neuropathy
7. Psychiatric problems
8. Lower sperm counts
9. Release of large proteins
10. Headaches
11. Delayed brain development
12. Immune system damage
13. Changes to hormone release
14. Interference with sexual development
15. Mucus membrane irritation
16. Motor weakness
17. Excessive hair growth
18. Lower sperm counts
19. Nausea/vomiting
20. Sensory impairments
21. Confusion

Sources

1. Paper bleaching (inc. milk/juice cartons)
2. Herbicides and pesticides
3. Manufacture of herbicides
4. Plastic bottles and containers
5. Garbage incinerators
6. Accumulated fish, meat, dairy products

ETHYLENE DIBROMIDE (EDB)

EBD is a heavy liquid with a smell like chloroform. This compound is usually mixed with carbon tetrachloride; please see that sheet as well. It gained a great deal of notoriety a few years ago when residues of this carcinogenic fumigant were found in foods. As a result, the use of EDB as a pesticide was banned in the US. The primary route of exposure is by inhalation of polluted air (e.g., contrails), although EDB can also leach from the soil into the groundwater.

Symptoms

1. Damage to the central nervous system
2. Nausea
3. Headache
4. Dilated pupils
5. Cyanosis
6. Circulatory failure
7. Respiratory failure
8. Reversible changes to the cornea
9. Weakened immune system
10. Irritation, rash, blistering
11. Dizziness
12. Vomiting
13. Diarrhea
14. Weak pulse
15. Unconsciousness
16. Liver damage
17. Kidney damage
18. Cancer in various forms
19. Damage to gastrointestinal tract

Sources

1. Insecticide
2. Lead scavengers in gasoline
3. Fumigants
4. Groundwater contaminants
5. Plastic protective clothing
6. Packaged foods like breakfast cereals
7. Dried fruits
8. Grains
9. Production of vinyl chloride
10. Rubber gloves

ETHYLENE GLYCOL

This is a clear, colorless, syrup liquid with a sweet taste, capable of absorbing twice its weight in water. By volume, it is one of the top 20 chemicals in production. The Federal Food, Drug and Cosmetic Act was passed in 1935 as a direct result of the deaths of many people after taking drugs sweetened with ethylene glycol, so this chemical is of historical interest.

Symptoms

1. Headaches
2. Irregularities to eye movements
3. Twitching of body muscles
4. Tightness of the chest
5. Shallow rapid breathing
6. Appearing drunk with no alcohol odor
7. Throat irritation
8. Eye paralysis and blurred vision
9. Rapid heartbeat
10. High blood pressure
11. Irreversible kidney damage

Sources

1. Antifreeze
2. Cosmetics, esp. with creamy texture
3. Ink
4. Automobile brake fluid
5. Urban air (low concentrations)
6. Paints
7. Glues
8. Polyester
9. Chemical solvents
10. Tobacco products

FLUORIDE

Fluoride is an oxidized compound of the element fluorine. There has been much work done in the last 30 years to suggest that fluoride is significantly more toxic that had previously been supposed. Some studies imply that as low as dose as 9mg could be fatal.

Symptoms

1. Arthritis
2. Chronic allergies
3. Can cause cancer
4. Immune weakness
5. Dilated pupils
6. Nausea, vomiting, commonly followed by diarrhea
7. Hypocalcaemia
8. Genetic mutations
9. Dental deformities
10. Non-cancerous tumors
11. Thirst
12. Headache
13. Abdominal pain

Sources

1. Toothpaste and dental products
2. Fluoridated drinking water

FORMALDEHYDE

Although known as a preservative, formaldehyde is also used in an enormous variety of other products and processes. One the most widespread is as a component of carpet and furniture finishes, which can off-gas for up to five years after installation. By weight, formaldehyde is among the top 50 industrial chemicals produced in the US.

Symptoms

1. Asthma
2. Candida
3. Chemical sensitivities
4. Crying
5. Food allergies
6. Depression
7. Burning eyes
8. Numbness
9. Cancer
10. Paralysis
11. Spaciness
12. Seizures
13. Conjunctivitis
14. Aching in the upper back and shoulders
15. Brain allergies
16. Chest pain
17. Dizziness, hallucinations
18. Mucus membrane weakens
19. Central nervous system disturbances
20. Hay fever
21. General malaise in new homes, stores
22. Shakiness
23. Rapid heart beat
24. Throat inflammation
25. Pollen allergies
26. Upper respiratory tract irritation, rhinitis, scratchy throat, cough

Sources

1. Resins and textiles
2. Air fresheners
3. Germicides and fungicides
4. Photographic chemicals
5. Cigarette and wood smoke, exhaust
6. Plywood and particle board
7. Ice cream
8. Insecticides
9. Artificial silks
10. Furniture
11. Construction materials, insulation
12. Cosmetics and shampoo
13. Dyes
14. Tanning and preserving hides
15. Toothpaste
16. Yeast/sugar beet production
17. Glass mirrors
18. Plastic bags
19. Foam and foam mattresses
20. Disinfectants
21. Explosives
22. Rubber latex
23. Plastic telephones
24. Embalming fluids
25. Cellulose esters
26. Waterproofing fabrics
27. Preventing rot, mildew and spelt in grains
28. Pharmaceutical drugs
29. Vaccines
30. Food preservatives

FORMIC ACID

A naturally occurring acid with a distinctive harsh smell that is produced by bees, wasps and ants, formic acid is found in the air, and also in certain fruits and vegetables.

Symptoms

1. Nausea
2. Increased nasal discharge
3. Throat discomfort
4. Blistering
5. Visual and mental disturbances
6. Severe acidosis
7. Diarrhea
8. Kidney damage
9. Breathing difficulties
10. Epigastric pain
11. Rhinitis
12. Intense thirst
13. Ulceration of all membranes and tissues
14. Circulatory collapse
15. Weak and rapid pulse
16. Clammy skin
17. Tissue irritation
18. Inability to speak
19. Ocular toxicity
20. Skin disease
21. Conjunctivitis
22. Inflammation and ulcerations

Sources

1. Paint remover
2. Airplane glue
3. Textile dyeing
4. Leather processing
5. Antiseptic in wine and beer brewing
6. Preservative in animal feed
7. Bare wires for soldering
8. Ant infestations

GLYPHOSATE (Round Up)

In appearance, this is a white odorless solid; on heating, it decomposes into toxic fumes that include nitrogen oxides and phosphorous oxides. Glyphosate solutions are corrosive to iron and galvanized steel. This substance can be ingested or inhaled (in aerosol form).

Symptoms

1. Brain fog
2. Ankle swelling
3. Respiratory distress
4. Hyperactivity
5. Irritation, rash, blistering
6. Pain in the feet
7. Burning eyes
8. Headache/migraine
9. Non-Hodgkin's lymphoma

Sources

1. Pesticides
2. Insecticides

GOLD

Traditionally the most valuable of the precious metals, gold is relatively soft and yellow in appearance. Apart from its monetary and trade value, gold is used in a wide variety of commercial and industrial processes and products.

Symptoms

1. Increase of blood esoinophils
2. Skin reactions
3. Bone marrow deterioration
4. Hepatic weakness
5. Gastrointestinal disturbance
6. Mild jaundice
7. Nerve conditions
8. Tremors
9. Aplastic anemia
10. Renal damage
11. Fatigue
12. Encephalopathy
13. Headache
14. Discoloration of mucus membrane
15. Deterioration of mental ability
16. Impaired coordination

Sources

1. Radioactive gold to treat tumors
2. Jewelry and luxury textiles
3. Dental work
4. Coffee filters

GRAPHITE

Graphite (or plumbago) is a soft, crystallizable form of the element black carbon. Graphite is metallic in appearance, though very soft. In nature, it is typically found in gneisses and schists, together with mica, iron oxide, quartz and other minerals. Widely used in the fields of chemistry, metallurgy, nuclear, and rocket science, it is known to cause allergic reactions in humans.

Symptoms

1. Stomach ache
2. Coughing
3. Black sputum
4. Ventricular hypertrophy
5. Dizziness
6. Graphite pneumoconiosis
7. Tissue death
8. Vomiting
9. Dypsnea
10. Bronchitis
11. Impairment of pulmonary function
12. Can cause cancer
13. Emphysema
14. Hardening of the blood vessels

Sources

1. Electrodes in electrical furnaces
2. Motor and generator brushes
3. Rocket motor nozzles
4. Metallurgical molds and crucibles
5. Resin-impregnated process equipment
6. Sporting goods: fishing rods, rackets
7. Charcoal and coke
8. Lead pipes
9. Meteorites
10. Anodes for electrolytic conversion
11. Sleeve-type bearings and seal rings
12. Missile nose cones
13. Linings for chemical reaction vessels
14. Carbon fibers in aerospace industries
15. Sail boats
16. Soot
17. Pencil lead
18. Old buildings with lead paint

IRON

Iron, a natural element that is also a magnetic metal, is not really a toxin; in fact, it is the lack of iron that is toxic to humans. Iron deficiency means lack of oxygen, wherever there is insufficient iron, oxygen will also be missing, and the impact will be seen in mental activity, the personality, and the nervous system.

Symptoms

1. Exhaustion
2. Lack of ambition
3. Fainting
4. Anemia
5. Listlessness
6. Melancholy
7. Nervous stress
8. Agitation and excitement
9. Inability to formulate plans
10. Insomnia
11. Turmoil in the morning
12. Acid reflux
13. Backaches
14. Migraines
15. Low energy
16. Dizziness
17. Nosebleeds
18. Poor recall
19. Depression
20. Lowered mental ability
21. Slowness of mind
22. Difficulties with studies or mathematics
23. Constant complaining
24. Disturbing dreams
25. Oversensitivity
26. Menopausal disorders
27. Reduced immunity
28. Toxic liver

Sources

1. Dulse
2. Dried fruits
3. Greens
4. Beans (especially black beans)
5. Egg yolks
6. Nuts
7. Chocolate
8. Kelp
9. Black cherries
10. Liquid chlorophyll
11. Beef
12. Gelatin
13. Coffee
14. Apricots, peaches, bananas

ISOPROPYL ALCOHOL

This organic solvent, also called "rubbing alcohol" is commonly found in pharmacies and in many manufactured products, such as cosmetics and supplements. It is frequently used in chemical sterilization procedures.

Symptoms

1. Unresponsive reflexes
2. Slowed and/or labored breathing
3. Low blood pressure
4. Can cause cancers
5. Dizziness
6. Drying and cracking of the skin
7. Personality changes (withdrawal, irritable)
8. Weakness in arms, legs: pins & needles
9. Low urine output
10. Nausea and vomiting
11. Reproductive dysfunction
12. Developmental toxicity
13. Changes in sleep patterns
14. Weakened memory/concentration
15. Confusion
16. Drowsiness, lethargy or fatigue
17. Hypotension, possible bradycardia
18. Gastroenteritis
19. Abdominal pain
20. Uncoordinated movements
21. Depression of central nervous system
22. Reduced coordination
23. Eye and skin irritation
24. Possible damage to the liver and/or kidney
25. Tachycardia
26. Ataxia
27. Possible hypothermia
28. Fever

Sources

1. Shampoo, hairspray and mousse
2. Cosmetics
3. Mouthwash
4. Shaving supplies
5. Vitamins, minerals and supplements
6. White sugar
7. Store-bought fruit juice
8. Making textiles and leather products
9. Car paints and spray painting
10. Printed circuit boards
11. Chemical packaging
12. Rubber weather strips
13. Furniture stripping
14. Used in printing processes
15. Carbonated beverages
16. Rubbing alcohol and alcohol swabs
17. Decaffeinated coffee
18. Cold cereals
19. Used to sterilize bottles
20. Bottled water

LATEX

Latex is a material derived from the sap of the rubber tree; it is used on a great variety of commercial, industrial, and household products.

Note: Cross sensitivity to latex is found in the following foods: bananas (high cross reaction), chestnuts, kiwi fruit, tomatoes, avocados, pineapples, apricots, grapes, papayas, passion fruit, cherries, figs, peaches, nectarines, plums celery, raw potatoes, and hazelnuts.

Symptoms

1. Rashes
2. Sneezing and/or runny nose
3. Facial flushing
4. Shortness of breath, wheezing
5. Anxiety
6. Feeling faint
7. Itching
8. Swelling/itching after medical/dental exam
9. Hives
10. Rapid breathing
11. Confusion
12. Shock

Sources

1. Rubber bands and hot water bottles
2. Condoms and diaphragms
3. Balloons and toys
4. Dishwashing or medical gloves
5. Shoe soles
6. Carpeting, rugs or rug pads
7. Air filtration systems
8. Bathroom/sink mats
9. Cosmetics
10. Diapers
11. Clickers and phones (buttons)
12. Anything with rubberized grips
13. Some mattresses and synthetic pillows
14. Sports equipment
15. Erasers and stamp pads
16. Weather-stripping
17. Sanitary napkins
18. Medical supplies and surgical fabrics
19. Parts for binoculars and cameras
20. Ziploc bags
21. Rubber galoshes and rain slickers
22. Elastic waistbands and yarn
23. Adhesives
24. Appliance electrical cords
25. Sink nozzle or stoppers, plugs
26. Cook top on stove
27. Dishwasher and/or fridge
28. Rubber tires of any sort
29. Some spandex, bathing suits, hose
30. Rubber nipples and pacifiers
31. Gym equipment and mats
32. Car interiors
33. Pool liners
34. Art supplies: paints, markers, glue
35. Newsprint
36. Slick ad inserts in newspaper
37. Hermetically sealed jars
38. Wheelchair cushions
39. Mouse pads, keyboards, calculators
40. Rubberized buttons

LEAD

Although its use is not as widespread as in earlier times, especially the 17th–19th centuries, lead is still common enough in many everyday products and processes. Children are especially susceptible, as a child's intestinal system may absorb up to 50% of an oral dose whereas adults will typically absorb only 5–10%. Lead is stored in the liver and bone, where it accumulates over many years. It can also affect the immune system and nervous system.

Symptoms

1. Madness (e.g., Victorian hatmakers)
2. Lack of willpower
3. Increased tooth decay
4. Renal degeneration
5. Destruction of bone marrow
6. Increase in diabetes
7. Behavioral disorders
8. Immaturity
9. Short attention span
10. Abdominal pain
11. Weakened constitution
12. Diminished ability to think abstractly
13. Allergic reactions to food/environment
14. Liver damage
15. Damage to spleen
16. Multiple sclerosis
17. Damage to central nervous system
18. Hyperactivity, impulsiveness
19. Cellular mutation
20. Lesions of the nervous system

Sources

1. Paints
2. Tin cans
3. Motor vehicle exhausts
4. Tobacco smoke
5. Metallic glazes
6. Water pipes
7. Insecticides
8. Gasoline and diesel fuels
9. Cracked ceramic glazes
10. Cracked lead crystal and glass

LINDANE (hexachlorocyclohexane)

Chances are that any chemical with a name this long is bound to be bad for you! Lindane is an organochlorine pesticide that is found in air, water and soil samples throughout the world. It has also been detected in human breast milk and amniotic fluid. In the U.S., it is still widely prescribed for treating head lice and scabies. It is a cumulative carcinogen and mutagen; it also has teratogenic, immunotoxic, and neurotoxic properties. In particular, Lindane affects the brain and limbic system, causing changes to the mood, affect, senses, and behavior. Lindane toxicity is particularly noticeable in those who are dieting, with eating disorders, and/or with low-protein diets.

Symptoms

1. Liver damage
2. Incontinence
3. Gastrointestinal disorders
4. Bone marrow problems
5. Aplastic anemia
6. Headache
7. Nausea
8. Fatigue
9. Seizures
10. Red/green visual changes
11. Precancerous and cancerous conditions
12. Grinding of teeth
13. Cyanotic circulatory collapse
14. Damage to kidneys
15. Testicular damage
16. Tachycardia
17. Anorexia
18. Damage to developing fetuses
19. Confusion, loss of balance
20. Hyper-irritability
21. Anxiety
22. Muscle spasms, abdominal cramps
23. Damage to central nervous system
24. Respiratory failure, pulmonary edema
25. Mental and motor retardation
26. Increased blood pressure, cardiac damage

Sources

1. Production of animal feeds
2. Wood preservatives
3. Milk, eggs, dairy products, some seafood
4. Car interiors
5. Prefab wood or concrete stairs
6. Canola seeds, plants, oil
7. Some fish, meat, flour, bread, onions
8. Shelf paper
9. Treatment of scabies and pediculosis
10. Tobacco
11. Used to control malaria, vector diseases
12. Pesticides on sugar beet, oil seed rape
13. Lice treatments
14. Chocolate with high cocoa butter content
15. Christmas trees
16. Pet/livestock treatments for lice and fleas

MERCURY

This is the only metal element that comes in liquid form: when pure, it is a dense, cohesive heavy metal. Not only is mercury used in a wide variety of manufactured products, it can also be found widely in the environment. In humans, mercury settles in the brain, kidneys and nervous system, where it causes neurological and behavioral disruptions, such as tremors of eyelids, lips, tongue, fingers, and extremities. It can be transmitted to unborn children.

Symptoms

1. Jerks and tremors, arrhythmia
2. Depression
3. Loss of vision, restriction of visual field
4. Fever
5. Loosening of teeth, sore gums
6. Nutritional disturbances, loss of appetite
7. Hypertension
8. Peripheral neuritis
9. Gastric disturbances
10. Brain damage
11. Abdominal pain
12. Need to spit a lot, drooling
13. Convulsions
14. Difficulty chewing and swallowing
15. Unexplained weight loss
16. Impaired memory or concentration
17. Ataxia
18. Allergies/asthma
19. Chromosome breakage
20. Deafness
21. Irregular heart beat
22. Kidney malfunction
23. Gingivitis, blue line at gingival margin
24. Metallic taste in mouth
25. Anemia
26. Marked changes of behavior
27. Fatigue
28. Skin eruptions
29. Nausea/vomiting
30. Colitis, acidosis
31. Pain in leg or breast
32. Reproductive problems
33.. Loss of sense of pain
34. Shyness, nervousness
35. Inability to speak clearly
36. Diarrhea, diuresis
37. Nerve fiber demyelination
38. Cerebral palsy

Sources

1. Hair dyes
2. Adhesives
3. Fabric softeners
4. Pharmaceuticals and supplements
5. Diapers and cotton swabs, cotton balls
6. Toothpicks
7. Batteries
8. Barometers and thermometers
9. Cosmetics
10. Water-based paints
11. Chemical fertilizers
12. Dental fillings, denture plastics
13. Bandages
14. Cigarettes, tobacco
15. Carpeting
16. Petroleum products

METHANOL (Wood Alcohol)

The presence of methanol is associated in 100% of diabetes cases with reproduction of pancreatic fluke stages in the pancreas. Chemically the simplest alcohol available, intense methanol contamination can lead to blindness. Methanol is frequently the result of home-produced liquor, and is therefore a serious consequence of alcoholic prohibition. Methanol is used in a wide variety of commercial and household products, as well as being a side-effect of certain mycotoxins and candida buildup. It is frequently used as a sterilizing agent in medical procedures. Long-term inhalation of the fumes may give rise to chronic toxicity.

Symptoms

1. Giddiness
2. Nausea and vomiting
3. Abdominal and lumbar pain
4. Cyanosis (blue skin color)
5. Damage to retina and optic nerve
6. Increase in uric acid
7. Chest pain
8. Peripheral polyneuritis
9. Sleeplessness
10. Fatigue, lack of drive
11. Mild psycho-organic syndrome
12. Symptoms of mild Parkinson's
13. Weakness
14. Trembling
15. Cloudiness of vision
16. Restlessness
17. Hyperglycemia
18. Acidosis
19. Central nervous disorders
20. Bilateral neuritis of acoustic nerves
21. Slowing of movements
22. Excessive salivation
23. Subjective pain at back of head
24. Link to diabetes and blindness

Sources

1. Sodas and carbonated beverages
2. Fruit juice
3. Artificial sugars
4. Baby formula
5. Fuel substitutes and additives
6. Cold cereals
7. Potatoes and potato skins
8. Sterilization residues
9. Store-bought drinking water
10. Regular and decaf coffee
11. Pharmaceutical drugs
12. Paints and varnishes
13. Gasoline antifreeze
14. Vitamins
15. IV treatments, inc. supplements
16. Powders stirred into drinks (even those labeled as health foods)

METHYL BROMIDE

This is an organic petrochemical solvent that is used in a wide range of products as a methylating agent. Methyl bromide can be ingested, inhaled, or absorbed through the skin.

Symptoms

1. Congestion of the liver, kidneys, brain
2. Insufficient circulation
3. Damage of the renal tubules
4. Severe headaches
5. Giddiness
6. Nausea
7. Tremors
8. Stuttering
9. Delirium, schizophrenic hallucinations
10. Confusion, lack of concentration
11. Sensory disturbances
12. Cerebral edema
13. Encephalitic lesions
14. Paralysis
15. Fall in blood pressure
16. Irritation, rash, blistering
17. Dyspnea
17. Bronchial edema and pneumonia
18. Epileptic-type convulsions
19. Prolonged cyanosis, with sweetish breath
20. Vomiting
21. Poor coordination, swaying gait
22. Feelings of drunkenness
23. Hypersensitivity of acoustic nerves
24. Visual and speech disorders
25. Sleeplessness
26. Motor disturbances, twitching
27. First to third degree burns
28. Vertigo and fainting attacks
29. Weakness
30. Hyperactivity
31. Numb extremities
32. Conjunctivitis

Sources

1. Fumigants
2. Fire extinguishers
3. Insecticides, especially on strawberries
4. Cooling fluid in refrigerators

MOLYBDENUM

This is an elemental silver-white metal that occurs chiefly in mineral molybdenite and as a by-product form copper ores. It is an essential trace element in soil, plants, animals and humans. Molybdenum is a good antioxidant to reduce the sensitivity of chemical smells.

Symptoms

1. Copper depletion
2. Changes to the central nervous system
3. Irritability
4. Lack of uric acid production
5. Dental caries
6. Cancer of the throat
7. Asthma
8. Bronchitis
9. Digestive disorders
10. Flu-like symptoms
11. High blood pressure
12. Insomnia
13. Muscle pain
14. Skin disorders
15. Water retention
16. Loss of taste
17. Liver and kidney damage
18. Unexplained weight loss
19. Irregular heartbeat
20. Sinusitis
21. Sexual impotence in men
22. Abdominal bloating
23. Body aches
24. Depression
25. Fatigue
26. Headaches
27. Hyperactivity
28. Joint pains
29. Poor concentration
30. Shortness of breath
31. Weak limbs

Sources

1. Buckwheat
2. Wheat germ
3. Soy beans
4. Cereals, whole grains
5. Vegetables
6. Radio, light bulbs
7. High-temperature aerospace applications
8. Dry powder in fertilizers
9. Pigments
10. Canned beans
11. Liver and other organ meats
12. Eggs
13. Cocoa
14. Alcoholic beverages
15. Electrical heating elements and insulators
16. Flame/corrosion-resistant metals coatings
17. Lubricants
18. Steel additive

NICKEL

This is an element and naturally occurring silvery metal used in a variety of products. The average person ingests 90% of nickel through food. There are no longer operating nickel mine or refineries in the U.S., but deposits in the soil from earlier years of operation represent a continuing source of nickel exposure.

Symptoms

1. Nickel contact dermatitis, like eczema
2. Chronic sinus infections
3. Intestinal cancer
4. Malaise
5. Capillary damage
6. Prostate cancers
7. Loss of sense of smell
8. Respiratory infections
9. Headache
10. Angina
11. Increased protein in urine
12. Depression
13. Sinus congestion
14. Low stomach acid
15. Nausea, vomiting
16. Mottling of teach and bone changes
17. Mouth cancers
18. Low blood pressure
19. Mult. brain, lung, adrenal hemorrhages
20. Lungs, nose, larynx cancers
21. Asthma
22. Allergic lung reactions
23. Decreased estrogen
24. Shortness of breath
25. High blood sugar
26. Liver disease
27. Low adrenal functions
28. Hypoglycemia

Sources

1. Hydrogenated vegetable oils
2. Paints, lacquers and varnishes
3. Nickel plated watches and spectacles
4. Oil and water-based paints
5. Many electrical components
6. Ceramic glazes
7. Metal glass frames
8. Metal smelters, waste incinerators
9. Medical implants, artificial joints
10. Spray paint
11. Nickel plating, cast zinc
12. Mordants in dyes
13. Tobacco smoke
14. "White" gold
15. Dental metal
16. Metal watch bands, jewelry against skin
17. Stainless steel implements, buttons
18. Accumulating in aquatic food chains
19. Batteries
20. Welding

NICOTINE

Although nicotine is a natural derivative of the tobacco plant and has been used by humans for centuries, it is one of the most toxic substances known to man. In the past, it was used as a pesticide, while tobacco was thought (ironically) to be beneficial for lung complaints.

Symptoms

1. Nausea and vomiting
2. Gastrointestinal reactions
3. Confusion, dizziness
4. Sweating
5. High blood pressure with slow pulse
6. Eye irritation
7. Depression
8. Peripheral blockage of breathing muscles
9. Excess salivation
10. Disturbed hearing and vision
11. Fainting
12. Hyperactive nasal disorders
13. Acute organ congestion
14. Renal hyperemia
15. Female genitalia pain
16. Seizures/Convulsions
16. Abdominal pain
17. Lack of coordination
18. Headache
19. Weakness
20. Atrial fibrillation
21. Tremors and restlessness
22. Diarrhea
23. Vasoconstriction and tachycardia
24. Insomnia
25. Mental confusion
26. Peptic ulcers
27. Pulmonary edema
28. Brain edema
29. Palpitations
30. Anorexia
31. Muscle twitching

Sources

1. Tobacco
2. Pesticides

OXALIC ACID

Oxalic acid (a calcium salt) is a major constituent of kidney stones.

Symptoms

1. Nausea and vomiting
2. Severe purging
3. Hypotension, cardiovascular collapse
4. Renal damage
5. Conjunctivitis
6. Irritation of respiratory tract
7. Increasing weakness
8. Vascular disease of the hands
9. Gastric hemorrhage
10. Brown discoloration of fingernails
11. Obstinate cough
12. Cracks and fissures in the skin
13. Tingling, burning, soreness of skin
14. Gradual unexplained weight loss
15. Burning pain in throat and stomach
16. Weakening pulse
17. Headache
18. Hypocalcaemia (low calcium in fluids)
19. Gangrenous skin ulcerations
20. Muscular irritability
21. Kidney stones
22. Inflammatory nephritis
23. Stiffness of limbs
24. Chronic respiratory tract inflammation
25. Severe pain in inguinal region
26. Slow-healing ulcers
27. Nervousness
28. Ulceration of mucus membranes

Sources

1. Contaminated ground water
2. Rhubarb leaves, spinach, edible greens
3. Brass cleaner
4. Rust removers
5. Hardeners for plastic dental molds
6. Inhalation of contaminated air
7. Auto products
8. Home maintenance products
9. Industrial metal cleaners
10. Freckle and skin bleaching products

PCBs or POLYCHLORINATED BIPHENYLS

PCBs look like yellow brown oils and smell like mothballs. Although manufacture and leaky uses of PCBs were curtailed in the mid 1970s; significant reservoirs remain in soils, sediments, water, waste disposal sites, and existing electrical capacitors and transformers. Exposure frequently occurs through consumption of water or contaminated foods, especially fish and possibly waterfowl. Poultry, eggs, and milk have been contaminated in the past. Like DDT, PCBs are extremely persistent in the ecosystem, accumulating in fatty tissues and along the food chain. PCBs can cross the placenta and inhibit fetal development.

Symptoms

1. Change in immune system
2. Respiratory distress
3. Liver damage
4. Abdominal pain
5. Grey-brown discoloration of the skin
6. Stillbirths, spontaneous abortions
7. Biliary tract, and gall bladder problems
8. Possible increased cholesterol levels
9. Thyroid toxicity
10. Acne
11. Skin rashes
12. Lethargy
13. Pigmentation of fingernails
14. Irritation of eyes, nose and throat
15. Jaundice
16. Nausea and vomiting
17. Fetal toxicity
18. May cause liver cancer
19. Weight loss
20. Dark urine
21. Male reproductive problems
22. Gastrointestinal weakness
23. Excessive eye discharge
24. Endocrine system problems

Sources

1. Transformers and capacitors
2. Detergents
3. Hydraulic fluids and lubricants
4. Adhesives
5. Carbonless-copy paper
6. Plastic parts subject to heating: TVs, radios, typewriters, even hand tools
7. Commercial soap
8. Insecticides
9. Inks and dyes
10. Protective surface coatings for wood
11. Fire retardants
12. Contaminated animal feed

PERCHLOROETHYLENE – 'PERC'

The Perchloroethylene group can include the following solvents: Tetrachloroethylene; 1,1,2,2-Tetrachloro-ethylene; Ethene, Tetrachloro-; Ethylene tetrachloride; Perchlorethylene; Perchloroethylene; Ethylene, tetrachloro- (TCE or PCE). Also called "perc", this organic solvent is universally used by drycleaners as a cleaning agent. It is strongly suspected of causing cancer as well as liver and kidney diseases. It tends to accumulate in body fat.

Symptoms

1. Can cause cancers
2. Liver damage
3. Kidney toxicity
4. Pulmonary edema
5. Eye irritation
6. Respiratory tract irritation
7. Dark urine
8. Lightheadedness
9. Dizziness and vertigo
10. Headache
11. Acute uremia
12. Conjunctivitis
13. Skin inflammation
14. Obstructive jaundice
15. Confusion
16. Delayed development in infants

Sources

1. Dry-cleaning
2. Chlorinated solvents
3. Aircraft manufacturing
4. Textile industries
5. Drinking water/vinyl coated pipes
6. Fatty foods adjacent to dry cleaners

PHOSPHORIC ACID

This colorless liquid is a nerve poison It is used in low concentrations to add a flavorful zing to some foods, including soft drinks. Perhaps that's how some colas got a reputation as rust removers. It is frequently used in the manufacture and refinement of chemicals such as hydrogen peroxide, ethylbenzene, ethylene, and propylene.

Symptoms

1. Nausea and vomiting
2. Dyspnea
3. Gastric hemorrhage
4. Rapid pulse
5. Scanty urine
6. Stomach ache
7. Dermatitis
8. Peripheral nerve damage
9. Gastric hemorrhage
10. Eye irritation
11. Pain
12. Circulatory collapse
13. Shallow respiration
14. Tracheal irritations
15. Pulmonary weakness
16. Nervous overexcitability of vagus nerve
17. Convulsions
18. Stiffness of limbs

Sources

1. Fertilizers
2. Soaps
3. Tang (food additive)
4. Cotton dyeing
5. Dental cement
6. Rubber latex used in extracting penicillin
7. Metal rust-proofing before painting
8. Catalyst in making ethylene
9. Livestock feeds
10. Waxes and polishes
11. Detergents
12. Tile cleaners
13. Water treatment
14. Flavor additive for sharp taste in foods
15. Manufacture of yeasts and gelatin
16. Manufacture of chemicals, e.g. propylene

PLATINUM

This element is a light-weight, silvery precious metal much used for jewelry and industrial components. The Republic of South Africa, the former U.S.S.R., and Canada account for nearly all of the world's newly mined or primary platinum-group metals. The kidney is the principal organ for excretion of most metals, as the number of nephrons provides a very extensive surface of endothelial cells for toxins to bind to, and the high blood-flow rate through the kidney enhances the level of exposure. Most refining procedures can be reduced to the metallic form from the chloride solution by the addition of ferrous salts or sulfur dioxide. Sensitive individuals will be affected by extremely small quantities.

Symptoms

1. Renal failure
2. Damage to skin
3. Urticaria of uncovered skin (e.g. neck)
4. Damage to gastrointestinal epithelium
5. Damage to liver and heart
6. Choking of adrenal glands
7. Depression
8. Blood vessels, tubular epithelial cells
9. Edema of the eyelids
10. Bone marrow suppression, depletion
11. Damage to the spleen
12. Peripheral vasoconstriction
13. Damage to testes and prostrate
14. Headaches

Sources

1. Automobile exhaust
2. Dental and medical devices
3. Electrical and electronic applications
4. Decorations
5. Powders, catalysts, colloids, compounds
6. Catalysts for fuel cells
7. Binary salts
8. Jewelry
9. Glass industry
10. Automotive catalysts
11. Sheet, strip, ribbon, foil, seamless tubing
12. Oxidation, staining, and electroplating

POLYETHYLENE

Ethylene is the hydrocarbon feedstock that is used in greatest volume in the petrochemical industry. It is a colorless gas with little odor. Polyethylene is used to make ethylene glycol, (used in antifreeze for cars), styrene (a component of synthetic rubber), polyethylene plastics (noted for their toughness and chemical resistance), latex paints and Dacron, Orlon, and rayon textile fibers. It is also used to make solvents, cellophane, and vinyl plastics. Polyethylenes can release vapors and gases which are irritating to the mucous membranes of the eyes, mouth, throat, and lungs.

Symptoms

1. May cause cancer
2. Damage to mucous membranes
3. Irritation to the lungs
4. Stinging eyes, nose, mouth and throat.

Sources

1. Unbleached grocery bags
2. Plastic food bags
3. Plastic pails
4. Kitchenware
5. Food containers and wrappers
6. Drinking glasses
7. Chewing gum
8. Milk bottles
9. Cutting boards
10. Garbage cans
11. Paper coatings
12. Heat-sealed plastic packaging
13. Electrical outlet safety covers
14. Coffee stirrers
15. Carpet fibers
16. Coated Paperboard Milk Cartons

POLYURETHANE

This name refers to a group of plastic materials based on polyether or polyester resin. The urethanes are block polymers capable of being formed by a literally indeterminate number of combinations of these compounds. The urethanes have excellent tensile strength and elongation, good ozone resistance, and good abrasion resistance. Combinations of hardness and elasticity unobtainable with other systems are possible. Polyurethanes are frequently used in textiles and foam materials, and therefore are frequently found in the home.

Symptoms

1. Irritation/inflammation of respiratory tract
2. Secondary infection of the lungs
3. Hepatic pain
4. Pharyngitis
5. Night sweats
6. Brain fog
7. Bronchial asthma
8. Pulmonary edema
9. Fatigue
10. Rhinitis
11. Carbon monoxide poisoning

Sources

1. Plastics
2. Medical catheters
3. Mattresses
4. Rug underlay, foam-backed carpet
5. Spandex fibers and garments
6. Orthopedic braces and splints
7. Sofas and other foam-based furniture
8. Automobile topper pads
9. Interliners/insulation in clothing
10. Certain glues and bonding agents

PROPYLENE GLYCOL

This colorless liquid is a nerve poison, solvent and coolant. It is widely used as a pesticide and as antifreeze; in fact, it was developed to take the place of the even more toxic ethylene glycol.

Symptoms

1. Raises osmotic pressure of blood
2. Sweat retention
3. Multiple endocrine problems
4. Metabolic acidosis
5. Edema
6. Skin irritation
7. Depression of central nervous system
8. Renal toxicity

Sources

1. Cosmetics, hair gel, soaps
2. Food additive in fruit juice
3. Diapers
4. Auto products (de-icer, foam, sealants)
5. Solvent for injections
6. Glass and surface cleaners
7. Citrus cleaners and degreasers
8. Antiseptic dressings
9. Liquid coolants
10. Theaters
11. Pharmaceutical preparations
12. Ready-mixed dessert toppings
13. Cleansing towels
14. Aerosol disinfectants
15. Fabric softener
16. Stain remover
17. Interior latex satin enamel paint
18. Water-based paints
19. Smoke in discotheques
20. Aviation emergency training

RADON

An element, radon is a colorless, odorless, chemically non-reactive radioactive gas formed when radioactive uranium and radium decay. Radon (and its decay products or "radon daughters") is present in the environment in quantities too small to be detected directly by the senses. Because radon is present in such small quantities, radiation detectors are needed to determine the level of their presence. Radon and its daughters often find their way into the lungs, either as gases or attached to fine particulates. In the lungs, two of the radon daughters are particularly hazardous because they emit alpha particles when they decay. Such particles can cause intense damage to the lining of the inner recesses of the lungs.

Unlike many other toxins, its elements are naturally present in rock and soil. Where we live and how we design our dwellings determine the dose we receive. Radon contributes to the problem of indoor air pollution; outdoors, it is sufficiently diluted by the atmosphere to pose a far lower hazard.

Symptoms

1. Fibrosis of the liver, hepatic cirrhosis
2. Immune system weakness/disorders
3. Pulmonary fibrosis, possible dyspnea
4. Can lead to sinus carcinoma
5. Spontaneous fractures
6. Can lead to lung cancer
7. Bone marrow disorders

Sources

1. Soil
2. Rocks
3. Mines and underground locations
4. Well water in some areas
5. Dust
6. Basements
7. Unventilated indoor areas

SALICYLIC ACID

This extract of willow bark is the main constituent of aspirin. It also turns up in a wide variety of fruits, vegetables, food products, and flavorings.

Symptoms

1. Headache
2. Ringing in the ears
3. Dimness of vision
4. Drowsiness
5. Thirst
6. Nausea and vomiting
7. Skin eruptions
8. Irritated mucosa and epithelial cells
9. Irritation to nasal passages
10. Acute inflammation
11. Restlessness
12. Pulmonary edema
13. Dizziness
14. Hearing loss
15. Mental confusion
16. Sweating
17. Hyperventilation
18. Diarrhea
19. Alternation in pH balance
20. Abdominal pain
21. Peripheral vascular weakness
22. Dehydration
23. Lethargy
24. Mental deterioration

Sources

1. Aspirin
2. Contaminated drinking water
3. Foods with natural salicylates: apricots, cantaloupes, dates, pineapple, grapes, oranges, raisins, raspberries
4. Dried herbs high in salicylates: thyme, paprika, garam masala, cumin, dill, oregano, turmeric, curry powder
5. Cosmetics
6. Theaters
7. Some topical creams and lotions
8. All organic, some inorganic, veg. soups
9. Processed foods /w synthetic salicylates: ice creams, gelatin, puddings, chewing gum, syrup, candy, drinks, baked goods
10. Flavorings high in synthetic salicylates: fruit, mint, wintergreen, caramel, butter, cinnamon, nut, root beer, vanilla
11. Ferret ear wash
13. Aviation emergency training

STRONTIUM 90

Strontium 90 is a radioisotope produced by nuclear fission, a substance that is chemically like calcium. Strontium is produced by reduction of the oxide with aluminum in vacuum. There are no commercial uses of strontium metal. It has been used to remove traces of gas from vacuum tubes. The most common source of contamination occurs when rain water is contaminated and subsequently taken up into grass, plankton, vegetables, and ruminant animals. As it is chemically similar to calcium, strontium then turns up in animal and human milk, as well as the bones of fish, animals, and humans. Strontium 90 is cumulative in effect.

Symptoms

1. Can cause bone cancer
2. Leukemia and other bone-related issues
3. Affects babies through mother's milk
4. Damaged teeth

5. Spontaneous bone fractures
6. Lumps on the bones
7. Weakened bones
8. Weakened thyroid and parathyroid

Sources

1. Atmospheric testing of atomic bombs
2. Food chain, through uptake by plants
3. U.S. Mail: irradiating all mail
4. Ship deck signs

5. Cow's milk from contaminated grass
6. Vegetables, plankton
7. Fish and animal bones

TBT or TRIBUTLYIN COMPOUNDS

Also called TBT or TBTO, these are metabolic poisons of very high toxicity. TBT is an environmentally damaging chemical commonly used as a fouling inhibitor in marine paint. Over the course of the 1980s, general awareness of the harmful effects of this substance gradually increased, and now it has been definitively proven that TBT disrupts the hormones of exposed organisms. These effects are particularly well documented in the case of the purple snail, but this highly toxic compound has also adversely affected oysters and larger mammals. TBT is one of the most poisonous organic compounds known to man, and the true extent of the damage to the marine environment ensuing from its use remains uncertain.

Symptoms

1. May cause cancer
2. Developmental toxicity/inhibition
3. Paralysis (in severe cases)
4. Diarrhea
5. Irritated skin
6. Flu-like symptoms
7. Respiratory or cardiac failure
8. Eye inflammation
9. Photophobia
10. Dizziness
11. Sore throat
12. Interstitial edema, white matter of brain
13. Reproductive toxicity
14. Neurotoxicity
15. Abdominal cramps
16. Nausea and vomiting
17. Difficulty in breathing
18. Inhibited metabolism
19. Progressive weakness
20. Nasal irritation
21. Headache
22. Visual disturbances
23. Coughing
24. Irritation, tightness or pain to lower chest

Sources

1. Paint ingredient
2. Manufacturing leather, textiles, wood
3. Controlling moulds, yeasts, algae
4. Antibacterial in damp areas (e.g. showers)
5. Residues in food
6. Industrial water systems
7. Certain plastics and coatings
8. Mothproofing
9. Latex spray point
10. Fungicide in exterior paints

TEFLON

Teflon is a non-stick plastic coating used in cooking pots and as a lubricant in many other household, medical, and aerospace products.

Symptoms

1. May cause cancer
2. Unexplained weight gain
3. Shortness of breath
4. Chills
5. Fatigue
6. Raised body temperature
7. Numbness/tingling in hands and arms
8. Coughing
9. Urinary, genital weakness
10 Spinal weakness
11. Flu-like symptoms
12. Tightness of chest
13. Headache
14. Sore throat
15. Malaise
16. Pulmonary edema
17. Common flu
18. Deadly to household birds

Sources

1. Medical implants
2. Cookware
3. Lubricants for bicycles
4. Remington SuperSmooth styling products
5. Uniforms and protective clothing
6. Bathroom and countertop cleaners
7. Stairmaster carpet treatments
8. Carpet protectors
9. Surface protection on floorings
10. Furniture and upholstery
11. Non-stick utensils
12. Heated appliances
13. Easy-care eyeglass lens coating
14. Paints
15. Sally Hanson nail products
16. Aerospace/aircraft parts and seals
17. Clothing protectors
18. Parts of many kitchen items

TELLURIUM

Tellurium is a naturally occurring non-metallic element, used in fabricating a variety of industrial products.

Symptoms

1. Garlic odor to all secretions
2. Suppression of sweat and saliva
3. Headache
4. Irregular perspiration
5. Pulmonary congestion
6. Disagreeable odor of the breath
7. Dry skin and mouth
8. Stupor
9. Cyanosis
10. Distinct fatty change of the liver

Sources

1. Glass
2. Photography
3. Nonmetallic element in electric rectifier
4. Components in the rubber industry
5. Certain alloys in the metal industry
6. Colored glass

THALLIUM

A naturally occurring non-metallic element, thallium is used with mercury. The actual mode of action of thallium has not yet been clarified. Possibly, like lead and mercury, it acts as a general cellular poison by inhibiting or blocking certain important enzyme systems, but details are unfortunately not known. The nerve fibers and the intestinal mucosa are particularly sensitive. Damage of the sebaceous and sweat glands may also be due to the excretion of thallium through these organs. Possibly some of the clinical symptoms are due to initial stimulation of the sympathetic nervous system. Thallium is cumulative.

Symptoms

1. Damage to nervous system and skin
2. Damage to cardiovascular system
3. Arthralgia (pain in a joint)
4. Insomnia
5. Mental confusion
6. Numbness/paralysis of legs and feet
7. Nephritis
8. Lymphocytosis
9. Loss of hair on body and head
10. Loss of appetite
11. Optic neuritis
12. Colicky abdominal pain
13. Obstinate unresponsive constipation
14. Restlessness
15. Tachycardia, increased blood pressure
16. Dry, scaly skin
17. Pigment at roots of hair
18. Semilunar white strips on fingernails
19. Hypotension shock
20. Swelling of the feet and legs
21. Damage to reproductive organs/fetus
22. Vomiting
23. Polyneuritis, severe pain in legs/loins
24. Angina-like pains
25. Wasting and weakness
26. Eosinophilia: cells that stain
27. Severe pain in calves
28. Albuninuria: serum protein in urine
29. Diminished sperm cell motility
30. Excessive thirst
31. Progressive dementia
32. Pronounced hypersthesis, soles of feet
33. Paralysis of peritoneal muscles
34. Inability to walk
35. Severe muscle atrophy
36. Early anhydrosis
37. Headache
39. Hypertension

Sources

1. Dental mercury amalgams
2. Rat poison
3. Toothpicks
4. Industrial poisons
5. Arctic, Antarctic thermostats
6. Dental floss

TIN

A naturally occurring element, tin is a soft, silvery malleable metal. It is frequently used in tin cans and other sheet metal alloys, as well as pesticides and some plastics.

Symptoms

1. Headaches
2. Seizures
3. Intracranial pressure
4. Liver pain
5. Hyperglycemia
6. Vomiting
7. Metallic taste
8. Motor and sensory impairment
9. Brain damage
10. Irritability
11. Coma
12. Neurotoxicity
13. Nausea
14. Abdominal cramping
15. Diarrhea
16. Gastrointestinal irritation
17. Chills and/or flushes
18. Accumulates in the brain

Sources

1. Processed foods
2. Plastics manufacturing
3. Toothpaste
4. Pesticides and fungicides
5. Dental braces
6. Industrial waste
7. Bronze and other alloys

TITANIUM

A naturally occurring element, titanium is a hard, silvery metal with a high melting point, much used in alloys. It was defined as an element in 1791. The commercial metal is produced from sponge titanium, made by converting titanium oxide to titanium tetrachloride, which is then reduced by molten magnesium. Because of its very low oxidation rate, titanium is used for aerospace components and sheathing.

Symptoms

1. Respiratory toxicity
2. Nausea
3. Reactivity in lymphocytes

4. Skin eruptions
5. Sinus conditions

Sources

1. White pigments, paint pigments
2. Hard metal facings
3. Metal castings
4. Plate, sheet, tubing, wire, forgings
5. Aerospace components/sheathing
6. Ceramic/glass pigments
7. Cutting tools
8. White rubber goods

9. Paper filler
10. Resistors for electrical insulators
11. Bicycle parts
12. Medical implants: joints, plates, screws
13. Dental braces
14. Cements
15. Toothpaste
16. Ceramic tile coating in sanitary apps.

TOLUENE

This is an organic solvent that is found in a wide variety of manufactured goods, and as a fuel additive. Toluene causes damage to unborn children; its toxic effects are exacerbated by alcohol, as this causes most of the toluene to migrate to the blood for maximum impact.

Symptoms

1. Dizziness
2. Nausea and vomiting
3. Irritability
4. Vomiting
5. Aplastic anemia
6. Impaired immune system
7. Dry skin
8. Depressed central nervous system
9. Kidney and liver damage
10. Insomnia
11. Tremors
12. Headaches
13. Euphoria
14. Paralysis
15. Depressed bone marrow
16. Multiple Sclerosis
17. Eye irritations, dilated pupils
18. Weakness and confusion
19. Extreme light sensitivity
20. Ventricular arrhythmia
21. Visual blurring
22. Rapid, shallow respiration
23. Disorientation
24. Depression

Sources

1. Gasoline additive
2. Model glues
3. Resins
4. Detergents
5. Lacquers
6. Perfumes
7. Saccharine
8. Exhaust from cars, trucks, planes
9. Evaporation from gas tanks
10. Vapor around gas stations
11. Arts and craft supplies
12. Paints
13. Adhesives
14. Dyes
15. Linoleum
16. Pharmaceuticals
17. TNT and other explosives
18. Oil and fuel spills
19. Cigarette smoke

TRICHLOROETHYLENE

This is a liquid that boils at 88°C; it has an aromatic, agreeable odor. Under the name of "TCE," it is today one of the most commonly used solvents in industry as it is noninflammable and possesses a high dissolving power. "TCE" is an organic solvent that is found in a wide variety of manufactured goods and is used as an anesthetic agent.

Symptoms

1. Irritation of the central nervous system
2. Paralysis of trigeminus (loss of teeth)
3. Disturbed vision
4. Degenerative lesions to brain and liver
5. Neurasthenic syndrome w/ forgetfulness, tiredness, insomnia, giddiness, headache
6. Peripheral neuritis
7. Tendency to fall
8. Hoarseness
9. Irritability, emotional instability
10. Burning of the eyes and hands
11. Loss of smell and ability to taste sweets
12. Fibrinomembranous gastroenteritis
13. Petechial hemorrhage peri/endocardium
14. Chronic brain syndrome: disturbed memory, thought, and affectivity
15. Frequent eczema of the skin
16. Feeling of drunkenness
17. Disturbances in swallowing
18. Paresthesia of the face and body:

Sources

1. Used as solvents for fats and rubber
2. Fire extinguishers
3. Dry cleaning
4. Varnishes, furniture
5. Used in glues
6. Degreasing metal parts
7. Synthetic resins
8. "Trichlorene" and "trilene" used in obstetrics for light anesthesia.

TUNGSTEN

A naturally occurring element, tungsten is a hard metal that is widely used in the metals industry and fluorescent lights. Tungsten is mainly held in the bones.

Symptoms

1. Pulmonary fibrosis
2. Respiratory toxicity
3. Bone disorders
4. Asthma

Sources

1. Alloy steels
2. Magnets
3. Grinding tools, high-temp applications
4. Electrical components
5. Fluorescent lights
6. Rocket nozzles
7. High-carbon steels
8. Radiation shielding

URANIUM

A radioactive metal element, uranium is primarily used for nuclear power and atomic weapons. It is the most common starting point for the production of usable isotopes. The soluble salts (fluorides, chlorides, nitrates, etc.) are rapidly absorbed by the lungs and can cause severe damage upon excretion through the kidneys. Uranium precipitates protein, which is probably responsible for its injurious effect on the lung alveoli, although insoluble uranium oxide is also retained in the lungs (on inhalation), where it causes radiation injuries. Most uranium is eliminated by the kidneys, where it causes severe lesions to the renal epithelia, particularly in the convoluted tubules. Uranium can also be deposited in the bones, where it takes the place of calcium; it is therefore particularly prone to crossing the placenta and affecting the unborn child.

Symptoms

1. Severe pulmonary lesions
2. Sense of suffocation
3. Obstinate dry cough
4. Pulmonary edema
5. Renal damage
6. Sever retrosternal pain
7. Dyspnea
8. Possible cancers from radiation effects

Sources

1. Nuclear energy production
2. Bombs
3. Production of various isotopes
4. Radioactive wastes

VANADIUM

A relatively rare metal element, vanadium is used to produce a variety of hard steel alloys and their associated products. Vanadium is toxic at relatively low doses and primarily affects the upper respiratory tract, brain, bones and kidneys.

Symptoms

1. Anemia
2. Anorexia
3. Diarrhea alternating with constipation
4. Headaches
5. Melancholia
6. Psychiatric disturbances
7. Manic-depression
8. Strong brain residue
9. Depressed bone marrow functions
10. Lung toxicity
11. Emaciation
12. Dry paroxysmal cough
13. Nausea
14. Urinary albuminuria, blood in urine
15. Vertigo
16. Fine tremors
17. Acute bronchitis
18. Greenish-black tongue discoloration
19. Red skin on face

Sources

1. Hard steel alloys
2. Handling dyes and dyed clothing
3. Candles (lit and unlit)
4. Cleaning boilers, furnaces, gas turbine
5. Gas leaks from outmoded equipment

VINYL CHLORIDE

This organic solvent is a gas at room temperatures. Also called ethylene chloride and chloroethylene, vinyl chloride is produced by reacting ethylene with oxygen from air and ethylene dichloride, and is the basic material for the polyvinyl chloride resins. These plastics were originally produced in Germany under the name of Igelite for cable insulation and as Vinnol for tire tubes. The most popular use for vinyl chloride is now PVC, which is widely used in plastic bags and storage containers, as well as synthetic furnishing fabrics.

In reducing exposure to vinyl chloride, the most important step is to avoid storing foods in PVC containers. It is illegal to sell these containers for the purpose of food storage, but they are available for other purposes. Do not drink liquids that have been mixed or stored in plastic pails or garbage cans. Ventilate new cars well before sitting in them: open the doors for a few minutes after the car has been sitting in the sun and/or leave the windows partially open while driving until that "new car smell" is no longer noticeable.

Symptoms

1. Can cause cancer from inhalation and ingestion
2. Mutagenic in animals and humans
3. Liver damage
4. Circulatory disorders
5. Feeling of intoxication
6. Lightheadedness
7. Abdominal pain
8. Weakness
9. Can cause cancer in liver, brain, blood, breasts and central nervous system,
10. Birth defects
11. Acroosteolysis (bones in fingers)
12. Lung complaints
13. Dizziness
14. Nausea
15. Slower response times
16. Headache

Sources

1. Auto dashboards
2. Plastic siding for houses
3. PVC pipes (plumbing, gutters)
4. New car interiors
5. Marijuana cigarettes
6. Tobacco products
7. Former uses include drugs, cosmetics, aerosols, refrigerants and anesthetics
8. Municipal water supplies
9. Alcoholic drinks and vinegars
10. Mineral water bottles
11. Oils and butter
12. Plastic packaging
13. Garbage bags and plastic trash cans
14. Plastic shrink wrap for cheese and cold cuts

XYLENE

This organic solvent is widely used as a chemical component of pesticides, plastics, and adhesives. It is the most acutely toxic of the common aromatic hydrocarbons, it travels up the olfactory nerves into the brain; this triggers the hypothalamus, which then causes malfunctions in the autonomic nervous system, limbic system, and vascular tree of the brain.

Symptoms

1. Cough
2. Nausea and vomiting
3. Feelings of euphoria
4. Giddiness
5. Ringing in the ears
6. Coma
7. Pulmonary edema
8. Slowed reactions
9. Depression or agitation to CNS
10. Restlessness
11. Contamination of hypothalamus
12. Excessive salivation
13. Trembling, tremors
14. Headaches
15. Vertigo
16. Confusion
17. Hoarseness
18. Irritation to eyes and nose
19. Poor balance
20. Unconsciousness
21. Resembles drunkenness
22. Limbic, autonomous malfunctions

Sources

1. Solvents
2. Pharmaceuticals
3. Paints
4. Nail polish and nail polish remover
5. Lacquers
6. Marking pens
7. Plastics
8. Pesticides
9. Paint remover/stripper
10. Air fresheners
11. Glues
12. Food processing

APPENDIX – TESTIMONIALS

TREATMENT FOR ANESTHESIA, VIRUS and STAPH INFECTION

All of my life I had a birthmark on the back of my head about the size of a quarter. As I grew older, the dermatologist thought we should have it removed as a precautionary measure. The dermatologist called the mark a "nevus sebaceous" and said removal was a common procedure. I made plans to have the procedure done.

The nurses prepared me for the procedure and explained how things would be done. A local anesthetic called lidocaine was used. I still had some feeling in my scalp after the 20-minute waiting period, so they injected more lidocaine into my scalp to deaden the area. After the area was numb, the doctor removed a football-shaped piece of my scalp (the birthmark was about 80% of the removed area). He then stretched the remaining skin together and stitched it closed. The scar is about 2_ inches long.

After the procedure, I was very light-headed and faint. My blood pressure and blood sugar levels dropped. Thirty minutes or so afterwards, I began to feel better. The days immediately following the surgery, I felt a normal amount of pain and discomfort. About three days later I had developed a lump on the right side of my neck. It was very tender and my neck began to get stiff. The pain in my head also increased and covered most of the scalp, not just the area worked on. The next day I woke up with a knot on the other side of my neck. I could not move my neck, and I had a great amount of stiffness in my shoulders. The pain all over my scalp was almost unbearable even though I was taking acetaminophen with codeine. My incision was not red or painful and it was not draining any liquid. I soon developed lumps at the base of my skull also.

I had been seeing Dr. Chernoff and receiving NAET for food allergies. She tested me for allergies to anesthesia, a virus and the staph bacteria. Not surprisingly, I was very affected by all three of these things. She treated me and warned me that my body would expel toxins for the next few days. Immediately following the treatment, my incision began draining blood, pus and yellow liquid for almost a week following the treatment. The next day I woke up with minimal stiffness in my neck and shoulders. I had no pain in my scalp and I did not need to take any painkillers. Twenty-five hours later I had no pain, no stiffness, and the lumps on my head and neck had diminished visibly. Five days later, the lumps had completely disappeared, and I still had no pain. My incision did continue draining for a few days.

In retrospect, I realized I had very negative experiences with the use of anesthesia in my body, local or other. I had not responded well to it in the past, and had taken much longer to recover from the use of it than normal. Discussing this with my mother, she also realized she had not had positive experiences with the use of anesthesia. She also developed similar lumps in her neck following surgery.

I did not have any expectations of the effects of this treatment. I knew that something needed to happen. The doctors treating me had no solutions except more drugs, and I knew that was not a good answer for me. This treatment took away all the negative effects of the surgery, and I believe helped heal my body much more quickly than otherwise. It saved me from much pain and discomfort as well as an infection in what appeared to be my lymph system.

Brianne, Albuquerque NM

I had a dental procedure done several days ago. I noticed that shortly after the appointment the lymph under my chin became inflamed. This pain lasted all night, and the next day nausea set in. That evening I had a beer, and thought that this was my problem. Dr. Chernoff diagnosed a reaction to anesthesia. In the past, I had four surgeries in six months and was heavily anesthetized twice. I did notice that afterwards word retrieval was extremely difficult and that my throat raced. So Dr. Chernoff's reasoning confirmed that my lymph swelling was directly connected to the anesthetic. Thank you for being so accurate, and being able to treat this problem long distance.

Margo, Santa Fe NM

TREATMENT FOR SELENIUM and CAR EXHAUST

If you suffer from asthma and allergies, this is a must for you to read. I want to tell you my story briefly and tell you that there is hope and a light at the end of the tunnel.

Fifteen years ago, I worked in a "sick building", and because of that I was over-exposed to mold and mildew among other things they couldn't even identify when they finally gutted and rebuilt the building. As a result, my immune system completely shut down. At first, the doctors didn't even know if I would live or die. As the first months went by, and for the next five years, I was treated with massive doses of steroids, eight allergy shots a week, and four inhalers four times a day. I started to recover, but was told I should file for disability and never work again. I was only 33 and couldn't bring myself to do it.

After three years, my immune system was built up enough so that I decided to go back to work. As health would have it, I would get a job and work for six months and then my system would collapse again and the next six months would be spent in rebuilding it again. Needless to say, I would have to quit the job.

Over the years, my asthma continued to get worse along with allergies. I become allergic to literally everything. I was sent to several doctors, including pulmonary doctors; they all told me I had to live with it – nothing could be done. I resigned myself to being lucky if I lived another five to ten years. My breathing and quality of life had gotten so bad, I wasn't sure if I even wanted to live (suffer) longer than that, despite the fact I now had grandchildren I wanted to watch grow up.

After meeting Dr. Chernoff, my life began to change. She was basically my last hope. I understood the principle behind the treatments and it made sense to me. But deep inside, I didn't believe anything would help.

She began treating me, and for the next year and a half, slowly the layers of asthma and allergies began to peel away. I now know that there is a happy ever after. I began at least having a fairly normal life. There was always the asthma and allergies hanging on, though (I have so many).

Last week, Dr. Chernoff treated me for selenium. I knew this was a biggy for me, but didn't know how big. After the 30-hour period following the treatment, my lungs were completely clear with no trace of coughing, pressure, pain or the other symptoms I have suffered for so many years. This was the first time in 15 years I felt completely asthma-free!

She then treated me for car exhaust. Walking alongside the road or being in the car as always bothered me to the point of getting sick. After the treatment, I no longer get sick. This was icing on the cake! This was the first time in so many years that I can walk outside!

Life is beautiful now. While I still have a long way to go, I have now seen the light at the end of the tunnel. Selenium turned the corner for me. If you have health problems, please don't give up. It may take awhile – for me it was over a year and a half – but you will and can have a good life.

Thank you, Dr. Chernoff. You have changed my life forever.

Joy

FATIGUE TREATMENT

Dr. Chernoff recently treated me separately for carbon monoxide and strontium 90. Prior to clearing for both, I had been literally fatigued, dim of mind, short of breath, insomnia-ridden and had hair-trigger irritability.

After the carbon monoxide treatment had cleared, I experienced a lift, but was still fatigued. My new work location for the past three months was the source of the strontium 90, and after the 40 hours of treatment clearing, I became totally alive, charging up the foothills, my irritability subsided, my sleep was restored and the environment was clear again in my eyes.

Huge thanks and blessings on you, Dr. Chernoff!

Sandra

CADMIUM TREATMENT

Everyone's worse nightmare is receiving a phone call that a loved one is in the hospital in critical condition. My father started with a sinus infection. Then he began to have severe vomiting. He was put in intensive care in critical condition with signs of cardiac arrest.

Fortunately for me, I know Dr. Chernoff. I called her immediately and requested her help. Dr. Chernoff found the problem and initiated a treatment for cadmium. Cadmium poisoning can cause vomiting and cardiac muscle problems. Within three hours of treatment, my father's situation was greatly improved and the doctors at the hospital declared the crisis time over.

I thank God every day for Dr. Chernoff. Life without her is clearly not worth living! Thank you, Dr. Chernoff, we love you!

Vai

NAET TREATMENTS FOR ACRYLIC NAILS

Dear Dr. Chernoff,

Please accept this letter as an appreciation of your healing talents.

Ten months ago, I injured my shoulder when I was lifting with my trainer. Over the course of the following nine months, I tried a multitude of things to heal my shoulder, including massage, chiropractic, and a topical homeopathic cream Traumeel. My trainer was also very conscientious not to irritate my injury with any exercise that would cause any shoulder pain. Not only did the above endeavors fail, my shoulder continued to lose mobility.

After going through the first five NAET treatments, you tested me for acrylic nails.

Wow!! I tested a definite YES for the nails causing my shoulder impingement!! Little did I expect such amazing results so quickly after my acrylic treatment. Within four weeks I am 95% improved.

My trainer is amazed at the fast improvement, especially, since he had to baby my shoulder during my workouts for nine months. Then, all of a sudden, within this last month we are now actually building my shoulder back up to what it was prior to my injury.

My continued education regarding wellness has answered my question of: "Did I injure my shoulder because of lifting too heavy a weight, or did I injure my shoulder due to my allergy to my acrylic nails?" Obviously, the NAET works!! My intentions have always been to be healthy and happy. Thank you for your part in fulfilling my happy, healthy lifestyle!

Affectionately, Julie

ACRYLIC TREATMENT

I could not believe that I was actually allergic to acrylic!

It all began with a period that wouldn't quit. I started bleeding the Monday after Easter. I had terrible cramps. Dr. Chernoff gave me several treatments: heart, iron mix, boosted progesterone. I felt better with each treatment, but I continued to have heavy bleeding, and I mean really heavy bleeding. I had big clots. I was afraid to walk down the hallway at work for fear that I would have blood pouring down my legs. I was wearing three pads at a time and changing them every hour. I even had to go home early one day from work because I soaked my pants.

I began to think that I was just going through menopause. I was just amazed that Dr. Chernoff said that I was allergic to acrylic. I have been wearing acrylic nails since 1985 (approximately 25 years) and I never thought that acrylic could be a problem! But I was willing to try anything! I was sick of bleeding and started to get scared because it was not stopping.

After being treated for the acrylic – I blew the treatment! I was devastated. Dr. Chernoff re-treated, and by 5pm that same day my bleeding started to stop flowing. I only changed my pad three times that day, vs. every hour! By Monday, I had just a little bleeding and by Tuesday, even less. I was down to changing my pads just twice a day. By Thursday I was just spotting, and feeling good, with no more cramps!

Thank you, Dr. Chernoff!

ALUMINUM TREATMENT

My son Jonathan has been seeing Dr. Marilyn Chernoff for Learning Difficulties. The seizures have been mostly controlled with medication.

The treatments have been beneficial – especially the last one. He was having trouble doing division. Weakness was identified with neuromuscular testing that his pituitary and pancreatic organ were associated with the problem. The culprit was aluminum. I just couldn't figure out where he was getting exposed to the aluminum since I eliminated all products in the household. We found that Topamaz, the medication he was taking for his seizures had aluminum in it.

Now after the session there is such a huge difference! Sometimes after a treatment, he will initially be better but then something else may arise. It has been some time since the treatment and he is now calmer, his whole behavior has changed. He has clearer thinking on just everything. Just amazing!

LaSonia

DIOXIN TREATMENT

I came to Dr. Marilyn Chernoff to clear some food allergies. During some of our testing, I mentioned a symptom of emotional paranoia, which Dr. Chernoff quickly linked to a chemical allergy. After she did some investigating, she found that the chemical was dioxin, a chemical found in meat and dairy products as well as the production of paper and cardboard materials.

After doing a treatment for dioxin, I was supposed to stay away from paper, meat and dairy products. I put on rubber gloves for less than five minutes, and the gloves turned a nasty color orange – you could see the toxins that my body was clearing. This goes to show how quickly and how the NAET treatments really work. Thank you, Dr. Chernoff, for the expertise and the care with which you have performed my treatments. After receiving these treatments, I am a whole new person!

Sincerely, J. D.

CLEARING ETHYLENE GLYCOL

I had just gone through three really big clearings. The clearings had shifted my body enough that some old problems were brought to the surface. I started feeling bad – low energy, sinus and lung congestion – so I made my 911 emergency to Dr. Marilyn. She discovered that I was reacting to ethylene glycol, which is used as a coolant in buildings and as an emulsifying agent in asphalt. It is manufactured in Houston, where I was exposed and my business actually has been selling it for the last 26 years. I am an avid runner, so I have been exposed to it through all the asphalt on the roads. After determining its uses, it was obvious that I had had numerous exposures, which would explain many of my complaints dating back to ten years ago. I felt bad throughout the clearing and for about three days my body was in detox mode. After that, I was back up to 100%. What a difference!

Elliot M.

TREATMENT FOR LYSOL

Dear Dr. Marilyn, my testimonial is long overdue. I have been receiving NAET treatments from you since June, 1998. My initial problem was a severe case of hives. Through the NAET techniques, you determined wheat to be the cause. I received relief immediately after the 25-hour period.

Since my initial visit, we have completed the eight major items in the food allergen group along with many bacteria, fungi and viruses. With each successive treatment, I feel stronger and healthier. I am able to eat different types of food without worrying about becoming sick with a headache. Additionally, this past year I have had less frequent cold-type illnesses. My immune system is stronger as well.

My most recent treatment is the cause for this testimonial. I had severe neck and shoulder pain for several weeks. I had several chiropractic treatments that brought minimal relief. Through your analysis, you determined that breathing something was affecting me. I use Lysol on a daily basis in our office restroom. During the treatment, I felt some relief and less tightness in the neck area. As the 25 hours progressed, I continually felt better. The clearing took several more days, but by the third day most of the pain was gone.

I appreciate your efforts on my road to health. Thank you and Dr. Devi for your continued efforts in NAET.

Sincerely, Dianna

CLEARING TEFLON

On April 9, 2004, I was feeling severe pain in my tailbone and surrounding areas. I also felt pain in my shinbones and the bottoms of my feet. I knew from experience that my sciatica and stomach were being affected. Dr. Chernoff checked me and found that I was reacting to the chemical Teflon, which is used in frying pans and utensils.

After the treatment, I had a huge sensation of release of tension in the tailbone for several hours as well as a constant itchy feeling, but all the pain had subsided substantially. I feel much better and plan to replace my frying pan and utensils! Thank you, Dr. Chernoff!

DEHYDRATION and POOR CIRCULATION

My symptoms consisted of severe dehydration, which was affecting my scalp. I would constantly drink water, yet still be dehydrated. My legs were weak, especially when walking, and I had poor circulation.

You treated me for an allergy to nickel. I avoided nickel for 29 hours and the difference in me is amazing! My breathing is better, my walking is better, the little stab in my right abdomen and my dehydration are both gone, my burping is gone, and my big veins are taken care of. I am a happy camper! Thank you so much!

Teri

RELIEVING BACK PAIN from ASBESTOS

The night before Dr. Chernoff treated me, I was sharing a hotel room with a colleague in Santa Fe, and couldn't sleep all night for the intense ache and burning on both side of my back about five inches above my hips. The next morning I nearly passed out at the breakfast meeting. I called Dr. Chernoff and she said it was not my kidneys (as I thought) but my lungs (where I had previously had two tumors, in 1973 and 1994). With the back pain, the problems were reactions to penicillin and asbestos. She treated me that afternoon for penicillin and the relief was immediate. The rest of the ache went away and I could breathe more easily and freely. It has now been three months since I was treated, and my breathing continues to be more clear and relaxed than it was before the treatment. The pain is completely gone. In fact, it's hard to remember how awful it was, now that it is gone.

Before she treated me, Dr. Chernoff asked if I had much exposure to asbestos and penicillin as a child. I can't be sure about the asbestos, but I grew up in LA in the 1950s, living in a house built in the 1920s. I also went to an elementary school that was probably built around the end of World War II, perhaps earlier. Years later, all such classrooms were remodeled to get rid of the asbestos. My memories of penicillin were more vivid. I got a fair number of shots as a child, because my father (who was a doctor) gave them to us when we had bad chest infections. Also, as a teenager, I was mistakenly diagnosed with syphilis and given large doses of penicillin every day for twelve days. I completed the full course of treatment before we found out that the blood test was incorrect.

Betsy

EYE PROBLEM CLEARS OVERNIGHT

Thank you for helping me with my eyes! And to think I almost didn't call and ask for your help!

I had terrible symptoms. My eyes were extremely itchy, crusty upon waking, yellow gunk was coming out, eyelids were swollen, and they continued to close up more and more. I went to the hospital and waited four hours until I could see a nurse. They didn't know what was wrong. They told me to take Claritin. If my eyes weren't better they would give me antibiotics. After hearing this I decided to try Dr. Chernoff.

Dr. Chernoff found that I needed a treatment for DDT residue. After the treatment, the itching stopped almost right away. By morning I was almost normal and now I have no problems!

Thank you Dr. Chernoff for all your insight!

Sincerely, Grace

Feeling Good and Need to Thank You!

I have always maintained what I believed has been a very consistent and active physical life, balancing my diet, work world, physical fitness, rest and spiritual life. My weight has ranged from 198 to 202 for about 25 years. On the other hand, throughout 2004, aches and pains began to escalate and I began to feel more and more sluggish, tired, mentally drained and at times a bit depressed. As I had not had a physical exam for over ten years, I scheduled one in early September 2004. All indications, including blood work, appeared that I should be healthy and feeling good. At the same time, I was commuting to work on my bicycle, 25 miles per day, and lifting weights as part of my daily ritual. Even though I was consistent, I knew I was not over doing my fitness activities. By October of 2004, my feet, which had progressively began to bother me, were burning by the end of the day. Each morning when I would get out of bed the burning and pain of my feet had me hobbling about and forced me to drive to work and change my daily routine. This was a serious set back for me as I have always been an extremely visible school administrator/educator. This foot problem shackled me to my desk, which began to drive me crazy. At the same time, I had previously scheduled another physical exam, this time as part of securing a life insurance policy. As I had these two issues going on, life insurance and my feet, I was also getting home every afternoon needing a nap, this was really sad for me. For my feet I began to see a doctor who recommended a cryogenic treatment for plantar faciaitis, which was to eliminate this foot pain with a three-day recovery period. Going into the surgery, my right foot was worse. Coming out of surgery my left foot was worse, the pain then began to crawl up my leg and my left knee, which had never ever bothered me, was now intolerable. This same foot doctor recommended a steroid-based prescription along with cortisone shots. During this same time-period, I was informed, by the life insurance company that I had failed the physical exam. It took a while for the blood test results to get to me but I had a 4.14 PSA reading. My afternoon naps went from 15 minutes to 60. This is when I decided that I needed to see Dr. Marilyn, who had been treating my wife, Joy, for several years with remarkable results.

Following my first session with you, Dr. Marilyn, the pain in my left knee was immediately gone, and the pain in my feet began to subside. Over the next few treatments, the problem with my feet is almost completely gone. At the same time, the treatments cleared my PSA problem with new blood testing showing a .9 PSA level. Dr. Marilyn, along with these significant improvements my energy levels have improved, my indigestion and gas problems have gone away and no more afternoon naps! I know that as I continue with my treatment plan that I will reach age 55 in great health, balanced and enthused about life! I have also recommended three individuals who each have shared with me their remarkable stories of improved health and elimination of pains - arthritis, and allergies. With your permission, I will continue to see you and recommend your services!

My sincerest appreciation for you and your God directed talents and energy. God Bless You!

Su Servidor,
Ricardo Dow y Anaya, Ph.D.

REACTION TO COBALT!

I had just traveled 3,000 miles from Florida to make a voice recording of a book for my metaphysical practice. I arrived at my friend's home in California where the recording was to take place. By the next morning, when I awoke, I found the glands in my throat to be swollen and a sore throat.

I immediately called Dr. Chernoff's office and left a message, regarding the glands and throat. I needed to begin voice recordings and I couldn't afford my voice to be impaired in anyway.

Dr. Chernoff got back to me, and said I was reacting to cobalt. I was floored because every bit of dishware, bowls, glasses, teacups, and serving dishes we had been using at my friend's house were ALL COBALT DISHWARE!!

I was cleared of the cobalt and my glands and throat returned to normal!! "Thanks, Dr. Chernoff for being a gifted medical intuitive and for saving my personal and professional life."

Vaishale

BIBILOGRAPHY

For those wishing to investigate the field of toxins further, the following provides a small but significant sample of the books/research available.

1. Brady, George S, *Materials Handbook*, published by McGraw-Hill, 1997

2. Casdorph, H.Richard, *Toxic Metal Syndrome*, published by Avery Publishing Group, 1995

3. Clark, Hulda Regehr, *The Cure for All Diseases*, published by ProMotion Publishing, 1995

4. Dadd, Debra Lynn, *Nontoxic and Natural: A Guide for Consumers*, published by Jeremy P. Tarcher, Inc., 1984

5. Dreisbach, Robert H, *Handbook of Poisoning: Prevention, Diagnosis & Treatment*, published by Appleton & Lange, 1987

6. Gittleman, Ann Louise, *How to Stay Young and Healthy in a Toxic World*, published by Keats Publishing, 1999

7. Goyer, Robert A, *Metal Toxicology*, published by Academic Press, 1995

8. Morelli, Jim, *Poison: How to Handle the Hazardous substances in Your Home*, published by Andrews and McMeel, 1997

9. Harte, John, *Toxics A to Z: A Guide to Everyday Pollution Hazards*, published by University of California Press, 1991

10. Hoffman, Gisela Kroeger, *Help One Another*, published by Hanna Kroeger Publications, 2003

11. Kirk, Raymond E, *Encyclopedia of Chemical Technology*, published by Interscience Encyclopedia, Inc.,1953

12. Mervyn, Leonard Thorsons, *Complete Guide to Vitamins and Minerals*, published by Thorsons, 1989

13. Moeschlin, Sven, *Poisoning: Diagnosis and Treatment*, published by Grune & Stratton, 1965

14. Peterson, Frederick, *Legal Medicine and Toxicology*, published by W.B. Saunders Company, 1923

15. Rapp, Doris, *Our Toxic World: A Wake-up Call*, published by the Environmental Medical Research Foundation, 2003

16. Rea, William J, *Chemical Sensitivity: Clinical Manifestations of Pollutant Overload*, published by Lewis Publishers, 1996

17. Steinman, David, and Wisner, R. Michael, *Living Healthy in a Toxic World*, published by Perigee Books, 1996

MARILYN CHERNOFF, PhD, ND, M.Ed

My biggest experience – the one that made the strongest impression in my life – was growing up in a rare and out of print bookstore in the heart of book row in New York City. Every room in my house had a library, including each bedroom. Our basement and garage had any type of book that one could dream of. My fondest memory was traveling with my father to purchase unusual libraries. One time we traveled to a house that had a lower level with rows and rows of thousands of books. It was like searching the great pyramid of Giza in Egypt (which I have also done) – delving in the mysteries of the unknown, to find that rare gem. It was at this house that my father purchased a rare set of books based on the hieroglyphics of one of the burial sites in Egypt; to my amazement, each of the three volume set was about 4 feet by 3 feet.

I was so impressed with these books that my studies led me into advanced Egyptian studies at Columbia University and Hunter College of the City of New York. I also became a certified educator, and as I worked with a wide range of children, I learned more and more about how people function, both physically and energetically. Over time, this combined with my innate medical intuition to draw me into the field of energy healing. After certifying in iridology naturopathy, botanical medicine and NAET, I now work with a wide range of conditions. My experience is that many physical ailments start with allergies and/or toxic sensitivity, which is how I came to do the research leading to this book.

EDUCATION:

Undergraduate:

- Egyptian Studies/Anthropology: New School for Social Research, NYC, 1965

- BA in Anthropology: Hunter College of the City of New York 1967

Post Graduate:

- MA in Education: University of New Mexico, 1969

- Botanical Medicine at Perth Academy of Natural Therapies, Australia, 1993, 1996

- Certification in Gifted Education: University of New Mexico, Albuquerque NM, 1970-72

- Trinity College of Natural Health, IN

    - Doctoral Degree in Naturopathy, 1996

    - Master Herbalist Certification, 1996

- PhD in Holistic Studies at Universal University, Clearwater FL, 2004

INTERNSHIPS in Iridology/Botanical Medicine

- Canberra, Australia, 1990, 1993 and 1996

- Perth, Australia, 1990, 1993 and 1996

- Dr. Ellen Jensen, Escondido CA, 1994

EXPERIENCE:

- Assistantship at University of New Mexico
- Five years teaching K-8
- 18 years specializing in gifted education

CERTIFICATIONS:

- American Naturopathic Medical Association
- Certified Traditional Naturopath
- Nambudripad Allergy Elimination Technique (NAET)
    - Member of the Board, National NAET Association
- Board Certified Alternative Medical Practitioner of the American Alternative Medical Association
- European Model Iridology, International Iridology Practitioner Association
- Certified as a National Biofeedback Practitioner

Dr. Marilyn Chernoff now runs a busy and effective healing practice based in Albuquerque NM with offices in San Luis Obispo, CA and Boulder, CO. A distance healer, medical intuitive and allergy specialist, she works closely with Dr. Devi Nambudripad, the creator of NAET, in broadening the applications of this innovative healing/clearing technique.

Dr. Marilyn Chernoff can be contacted at 877-222-9146 or at The Healing Center, 1924 Juan Tabo, Suite A, Albuquerque NM 87112 at 505-292-2222, email: dr.marilyn@earthlink.net.

ISBN 1-41206422-8